TWO ASPIRIN – SECOND DOSE

by John N. Withers, MD, FACS

IPO PUBLISHING COMPANY
P.O. Box 1490
Kahului, Maui, Hawaii 96732

International Standard Book Number: 0-9624722-1-2

Library of Congress Catalog Card Number: 90-083740

Withers, MD, FACS, John N.

Two Aspirin – Second Dose

A collection of fifty articles covers a wide variety of medical concerns. Articles provide information and advice about medical problems in a style that is interesting and easy to understand by a non-medically oriented audience. Index. 129 pages.

Published and Distributed by   Ipo Publishing Company
P.O. Box 1490
Kahului, Maui, Hawaii, USA 96732

To the memory of Bill Kohne
a father
an attorney
a community leader
a friend

DISCLAIMER

The purpose of this book is to educate and entertain the reader regarding certain medical topics which may have a bearing on his/her health. This book is not to be used as a "self-diagnosis" or a "self-treatment" book. It is not to replace visits to the appropriate physicians when they are indicated. The reader may worsen his condition if unnecessary delay occurs. The author, any co-writers, editors and publishers of this book shall have neither liability nor responsibility to any person or entity with respect to any loss or damage caused or alleged to be caused directly or indirectly by the information contained in this book.

TABLE OF CONTENTS

INTRODUCTION

A year has passed since the publishing of *TWO ASPIRIN –
FIRST DOSE*. The wonderful, positive response from readers has
encouraged me to devote my time to compiling another 50 articles
for *TWO ASPIRIN – SECOND DOSE*. The source of these articles
is my weekly medical column in *The Maui News*.

It is very important that patients, as well as doctors, keep up-
to-date on new developments in medicine. New methods of treatment are reported in the newspapers and on television daily. As a
physician, I am constantly reading and learning new ways to treat
old diseases. Since my years as a surgical resident, I have seen the
treatment of breast cancer evolve from the sacrosanct radical
mastectomy (removal of the breast and the underlying muscles) to
the modified radical (not removing the muscle), and then to the
"lumpectomy" (removing just the cancerous lump). There have
been many examples through the years where doing less has
proved to be better.

It is equally important for individuals to keep abreast of
changes in medicine to be sure that their doctors are "keeping up."
But how can a non-medical person learn without being bored to
tears and falling asleep after the first page in a medical book?
Certainly, everyone should have a medical reference book on
hand, and an excellent one is *The American Medical Association
Family Medical Guide*, published by Random House. While very

thorough, *The Guide* is not a book that you would select for enjoyable evening reading and get a laugh or two while learning some medical facts.

In contrast, I have attempted to make my articles interesting as well as educational. Making them clear and understandable was another matter and I relied upon my wife's assistance in proof-reading. Carole would circle the medical terms with a red pen and ask, "What do you mean by this?" or "Can't you say this better?" I want to thank Victor C. Pellegrino, author and teacher at Maui Community College, for help in editing and publishing both TWO ASPIRIN books. Lauren Hogan, a close family friend, deserves special thanks for the final editing. Thanks also goes to Cheryl J. KauhaaPo of *Just Your Type*, for composition and layout.

Your family doctor is essential in maintaining your health. This book is not meant to replace his care but rather to give you more information to work with him. When medical problems arise, see your physician right away. If it is nothing serious, and he is out playing golf, then "Take two aspirin, go to bed, and call him in the morning."

1 Medications

ASPIRIN – 1990

Another benefit from aspirin has been found! *The New England Journal of Medicine* (3-22-90) reports that one aspirin a day reduced the rate of ischemic strokes by 50% in patients under age 75 who had atrial fibrillation! Atrial fibrillation is the condition when the upper chambers of the heart fail to contract (beat), which allows the blood to pool in the chambers and form clots. If a clot breaks free from the heart, it may be carried by the blood stream to the brain where it will finally lodge in a small vessel and cause a stroke. This type of stroke occurs in the U.S. every year to 75,000 people. Recently, 1,224 patients with atrial fibrillation were studied at 20 hospitals and medical schools. They were treated with aspirin, warfarin (a blood thinner) or a placebo (a sugar pill). After one year, because it was obvious that aspirin reduced the rate of ischemic strokes (strokes from blood clots) by 50%, the use of sugar pills was discontinued; the study is still being continued to compare the benefits and risks of aspirin vs. warfarin (the blood thinner).

Aspirin, or acetylsalicylic acid (ASA), was first compounded by The Bayer Company of Germany in 1899. It was a great improvement over salicylic acid which had been used since ancient Greece when Hippocrates had his feverish patients chew on the bark of a willow tree (which contains salicylic acid). Since 1899, aspirin has become so successful and widely used, that it is now the standard against which new medications are evaluated.

Three common uses of aspirin are to reduce pain, to lower a fever, and to treat arthritis. Doctors refer to these properties as analgesic (against pain), antipyretic (against fever), and anti-inflammatory (against swelling).

Within the last ten years, aspirin's ability to delay clotting of the blood has been studied at great length. This property has been not only a benefit, but has also been aspirin's greatest danger. It occurs because aspirin prevents the microscopic blood platelets from sticking to each other, which is the start of a blood clot. This is a benefit if the doctor is attempting to reduce the recurrence of a heart attack or thrombophlebitis (blood clots) in the legs. But it is a danger if the patient has a bleeding ulcer along with the arthritis the doctor is trying to treat.

The FDA (Federal Drug Administration) has approved the professional labeling of aspirin "to reduce the risk of death and/or non-fatal myocardial infarction (heart attack) in patients with a previous infarction or unstable angina pectoris (heart pains)." A single buffered aspirin a day is the recommended dose.

Aspirin provides an inexpensive way to reduce heart attacks if the patient is already having trouble, but what about those who have not yet had problems? Would routine use of aspirin reduce the risk of a heart attack? Dr. Charles Hennekens of Harvard Medical School studied this question with the help of 22,071 healthy "guinea pig" doctors across the U.S. For six years, each doctor took a "white pill" every other day. One-half of the doctors took a buffered aspirin, while the other half swallowed a placebo (sugar pill). In 1988, at the completion of the study, it was learned that the doctors taking an aspirin every other day had only half the rate of heart attacks as did those taking the placebo! I learned that I had been taking the aspirin, and I am continuing this practice.

The recommendation at the completion of the study was that "healthy" men, 40 years or older, should consider taking an aspirin every other day but ONLY AFTER CONSULTING WITH THEIR PHYSICIAN.

On the other side of the coin are the dangers associated with the use of aspirin. Some people will develop rashes and a rare person will have an anaphylactic reaction (collapse in shock) upon taking it. Gastritis (severe stomach irritation), ulcers, bleeding during surgery, and increased sensitivity to coumadin (a blood thinner) are all dangers of aspirin use. Pregnant women should avoid aspirin during the final weeks of pregnancy and patients should avoid it the week prior to elective surgery.

The Surgeon General has strongly advised that children and teenagers not be given aspirin during infections of influenza or chicken pox because of the possibility of developing Reye's Syndrome, a rare but possibly fatal disease.

Aspirin remains a very important drug, especially for men over 40. I hope you have a better understanding of its use when your doctor says, "Take two aspirin, go to bed and call me in the morning."

DECAFFEINATED COFFEE:
To Use or Not to Use

No wonder the public is angry with the medical profession. We have taken away most of the pleasures in life. First to go were smoking and being a lazy couch potato. Next were eating red meats, ice cream, eggs, coconut pies and drinking regular coffee. The American public was finally exercising regularly, watching its cholesterol and drinking decaffeinated coffee. Then medical researchers announced on TV that decaffeinated coffee might actually INCREASE a person's cholesterol! What will be next to go?

While enjoying several cups of decaffeinated coffee in the morning, I did some reading to determine if decaf coffee might be dangerous to my health, and to learn how it was processed.

The reports show that the health risks of caffeine in coffee are that it can speed up the heart rate, produce tremor and cause insomnia. For a short time there was concern that cancer of the pancreas might in some way be associated with drinking coffee, but that view has now been discredited.

The average cup of coffee contains about 100 milligrams of caffeine and the decaffeinating processes removes about 97% of it. For comparison, a "strong" cup of tea or a 12 ounce can of cola has about 50 milligrams of caffeine.

There are four commonly used processes to extract the caffeine from the green coffee bean before roasting. The first, and oldest, is to steam the beans, which brings the caffeine to the surface, and then soak them in a solvent which dissolves the caffeine. Next, the resultant batch is treated again with steam which boils off the solvent with the caffeine. The worry of the consumer is whether or not any of the solvent, methylene chloride, remains on the bean, and whether or not it is dangerous to ingest. The producers claim that all of the solvent is removed by the final stage of roasting at 400° F, while the FDA (Federal Drug Administration) believes that methylene chloride is not cancer producing.

With the public wanting to drink as few "chemicals" as possible, other methods for decaffeinating coffee have been developed.

The second method is to soak the beans in water which removes the caffeine but many of the flavors also. The water is separated from the beans and then treated with a solvent to dissolve the caffeine. Next the water is boiled to remove the solvent and caffeine, and returned to the beans with the original flavors. These solvents are what worries the consumer.

The third method is "the Swiss water process" which again soaks the beans in water. Instead of using solvents, the water is passed through an activated charcoal filter to remove the caffeine. The consumer is usually more receptive to this process because it uses no "chemicals" and is considered "natural."

The most recently developed method for extracting caffeine from the coffee bean is the use of "supercritical" carbon dioxide. As carbon dioxide is constantly being made by our bodies and removed by the lungs, it is considered "safe" by consumer groups. In this process, the carbon dioxide is heated to 40-80° C and pressurized to 1740-2610 psig. The supercritical carbon dioxide selectively removes the caffeine, leaving behind the bean components responsible for the coffee's aroma and flavor. Unfortunately, the process is very expensive, but several major brands are being processed this way.

The can containing my morning decaf coffee states, "The Colombian coffee beans are decaffeinated with natural elements utilizing a patented European process to gently remove the caffeine." Considering that the beans for my morning cup have traveled from Colombia, South America to Switzerland, then to the Mainland and finally to Hawaii, I should take more time to enjoy its flavors. Then again, how can one decide which brand and process is perfect?

You can learn which method is used to produce your favorite brand of decaffeinated coffee. The labels on the cans are very vague, however, and filled with pleasing phrases such as "natural" processes. Several brands give 800 telephone numbers to call, so I did. Their answers were interesting: Sanka and decaffeinated

Yuban, both made by General Foods, are produced using carbon dioxide; however, decaffeinated Maxwell House, also a General Foods product, is made using ethyl acetate, a naturally occurring solvent found in fruits.

In the final analysis, individuals will have to decide which coffee to choose depending upon their own taste buds and their likes of dislikes for certain flavors. Today, all methods for decaffeinating coffee are considered safe.

Regarding the risk of decaffeinated coffee increasing your cholesterol, the studies are very conflicting and confusing. The safest approach is to drink it in moderation, to avoid other foods with cholesterol and saturated fats, and to exercise daily.

SUNSCREENS

"Play Now, Pay Later"is the slogan of the American Cancer Society in its campaign against skin cancer caused by exposure to the sun. Several of my patients, with their red blotchy faces, are walking proof of this warning.

It takes 20 to 40 years of intermittent exposure to the sun before skin cancer occurs, but when it does, others will follow. Not only does the sun destroy the cells on the top of the skin, but it also penetrates deeper into the skin and destroys the elastic tissue. This results in wrinkles on the exposed body areas, such as the face, neck, or the back of the hands.

The actinic (sun) changes are gradual and progress from normal skin to actinic keratosis (small roughened areas) to skin cancer (squamous cell and basal cell cancers.) This is most common among blue eyed, fair skinned individuals. It becomes rarer among darker skinned people. If nothing is done to stop this progression, then multiple small operations will become necessary to remove these cancers.

Recently a new method has been found to treat the actinic keratosis before it changes into the final stages of skin cancer. This is the application of Efudex cream to exposed areas which may be harboring the actinic keratosis changes. Efudex cream contains 5-fluorouracil which is a drug that is used to help destroy different cancers in the body, such as breast and colon cancers. It works by interfering in the synthesis of DNA in rapidly dividing cells (as in cancers). The medication acts only on the skin which has developed the actinic keratosis, but does not affect the normal skin.

The cream is applied twice a day for two to three weeks to skin that is exposed to the sun, particularly the face, ears, backs of hands and the shoulders. By the end of the first week the areas that contain actinic changes will show a blotchy redness. By the end of the second week these areas will be bright red and painful, evidence that the actinic keratosis is being destroyed. All my patients are amazed at the amount of unsuspected damage the sun has already caused. After the treatment is stopped, the redness subsides and new skin gradually covers the areas of the old keratosis.

Until 15 years ago the only way to avoid skin cancer was to stay indoors for your lifetime. Today, many of us old-timers have already had a healthy dose of the sun's rays and will probably develop several skin cancers. Fortunately, this need not be the case for younger adults and children. With the introduction of the "sunscreen" creams, people today can enjoy the sun, obtain a controlled tan and protect their skin.

According to *Consumer Reports* the different sunscreens are similar and vary only in their SPF (sun protection factor) ratings and their prices. The SPF is the multiple of the time necessary to produce a given change in the skin. If it normally takes you 30 minutes to get "pink", a sun-block of SPF 10 would allow you five hours in the sun before you would have the same damage (or color) to your skin.

My advice to the young and old is to use sunscreen faithfully. If it takes 30 years to develop skin cancer, then a sun-block of SPF 15 will protect you until you are 450 years old! Happy sunning! Good-by skin cancer!

STEROIDS

"Doctor, what do you mean you are going to order a steroid cream for my rash? Will I grow hair and develop muscles? Will I be arrested for using steroids?" What is the poor patient to do in these days of "drug testing" and the "abuse" of steroids? It is time for some education on the use and abuse of steroids.

Steroids are divided into two major categories: adrenocortical steroids, occurring in the adrenal gland (a small gland that sits on top of each kidney), and androgenic steroids, produced mainly by the testicles.

Adrenocortical steroids are extremely important in medicine and have definite uses and dangers. The major benefit stems from their ability to reduce and inhibit the inflammatory process. In conditions such as arthritis, ulcerative colitis (an inflammation of the bowel), and hepatitis (an inflammation of the liver) there will be an inflammatory response with swelling, increased white cells, and fibrin deposition (which causes scarring). Adrenocortical steroids are the "miracle drugs" shown to reduce and stop this response. Modern treatment of arthritis, carditis (an inflammation of the heart), and ulcerative colitis would be impossible without this type of steroid medication.

There are dangers, however, when using these drugs. The "side-effects" or dangers of adrenocortical steroids are very serious. Increased infections, bleeding ulcers of the stomach and duodenum, cataracts, osteoporosis and fractures of the back are just a few of the complications that accompany prolonged use. Although adrenocortical steroids can save lives, they must be used with care and not be abused.

The second category of steroids is the androgenic steroids. These are the ones causing all the fuss among athletes that we have heard and read about. In the body most of these steroids are produced by the testicles in the male, but small amounts can be made by the ovaries and the adrenal glands. Their actions in the normally developing boy are to increase the musculature, increase height, and develop masculine hair patterns.

Because of the normal response of increasing musculature, weight-lifters, body-builders and athletes have used excessive amounts in their search for increased strength. As a result, many abuses and complications have occurred. Decreased sperm counts, hepatitis (liver inflammation), psychosis (mental illness), and increased injuries have been seen in individuals using excessive amounts of androgenic steroids. There are concerns about an increase in cases of liver cancers and heart attacks, but these worries have not yet been confirmed.

Because of these detrimental effects, androgenic steroids were first banned by amateur sport organizations, such as the Olympics and NCAA, and more recently by professional organizations, such as the NFL. However, a number of top athletes have already been injured or expelled. Oklahoma University's Brian Bosworth was barred by the NCAA from playing in the Orange Bowl on January 1, 1987, because he tested positive for using androgenic steroids. He claimed that he was given the drugs by a physician for a "knee injury." The doctor was never identified and you now know (from reading the above information) that adreno-cortical steroids, not androgenic steroids, are used for reducing the inflammation in knee injuries. In 1988, Bosworth suffered numerous injuries while playing for the Seattle Seahawks. Whether or not his "muscle mass" is too large for his frame is a matter of conjecture.

The 1988 Olympics in Korea will be remembered for many exciting events and beautiful programs. It will also be remembered for the expulsion of Ben Johnson and the loss of his gold medal for the 100 meter dash when he was discovered to have taken androgenic steroids.

A frightening story by Tommy Chaikin, a lineman for South Carolina University, was reported in *Sports Illustrated,* (10-24-88). In trying to increase his weight, muscle mass and strength, he got "hooked" on androgenic steroids. His coaches were happy when his weight went from 210 to 260 pounds and his strength in bench pressing increased from 300 to 500 pounds. Unfortunately, he also developed hepatitis, aggressiveness, hostility, and severe depression. He hit the bottom when he attempted suicide by holding a gun to his head. He was stopped by his friends, and has since received therapy and stopped using the drug.

A *U.S. News & World Report* (12-26-88) survey estimates that 1 in 15 young Americans uses "steroids" to improve appearance or strength. This is shocking! The dangers that are already known and those that are feared should make parents and coaches realize that users are risking terrible complications for a very short-term gain. God gave each of us our own body. We can improve on it with exercise and a proper diet, or we can destroy it with drugs for the "quick fix."

NICOTINE ADDICTION

Which country is exporting billions of dollars of an addicting drug, causing thousands of deaths in other countries? You say, Colombia? Yes, but to an even greater extent, the United States! It is certainly hypocritical that we spend millions of dollars to fight the importation of cocaine, while at the same time our government encourages the exportation of cigarettes to Japan and Southeast Asia.

Dr. John Slade, speaker at the Hawaii Medical Association's Annual Meeting, revealed these startling facts. Considered an expert in the field of drug addiction and its treatment, many of his statements on cigarettes and nicotine addiction were new and thought provoking.

While the Public Health Service estimated that 390,000 Americans died in 1985 as a direct result of smoking cigarettes, it is believed that 2.5 million people died world-wide because of this habit! Fortunately, use is declining in this country, but U.S. production is *increasing* because we are exporting more to countries around the world.

Nicotine addiction is considered every bit as strong as cocaine or heroin. A sad statistic is that 50% of nicotine addicts are hooked BY THE AGE OF 13! Most adults who smoke say they would like to quit. Many try, but few succeed. The common course is to quit for several weeks or months, suffer a relapse, and quit again. After many attempts, success may be achieved with the help of the family and the family physician.

Dr. Slade challenged the primary care physicians to treat the disease of nicotine addiction with as much enthusiasm as they treat the diseases of diabetes or hypertension (high blood pressure). Certainly, nicotine addiction kills as many people as do these other two diseases. Two books helpful in quitting smoking, which were recommended by Dr. Slade, are: *Freedom from Smoking for You and Your Family* from the American Lung Association, and *If Only I Could Quit* by Karen Casey.

Cigarette smoking has been the most deadly epidemic of the 20th century. By the 1950's, even the tobacco companies began to admit that "there might be" something harmful in cigarettes. Filtered and "low tar" brands were introduced in an attempt to appease the public's fears. One of the early "filters" contained asbestos! Today 99% of the cigarettes sold are "filtered" and 50% are "low tar." However, as the addicting chemical is nicotine, and if the filter cuts down on the nicotine from each cigarette reaching the person's lungs, he/she must smoke more cigarettes to reach the desired nicotine "high."

I am sure that most nonsmokers would agree with me that the air is nicer to breathe now that smoking is restricted in public buildings and more airplane flights. Dr. Slade pointed out that even nonsmokers absorb tobacco smoke when they are confined to areas where smoking is permitted. Many studies have shown that nonsmoking spouses of smokers have a higher risk of cancer than normal. Yes, smokers have their rights—as long as they don't exhale.

Tobacco has been grown in America for centuries, but we are only now discovering its addiction and dangers. With the strong winds blowing against the tobacco industry, hopefully by the end of the next century we can have a "smoke free society" both here and abroad.

2 Health Habits

BROCCOLI AND GEORGE

"Georgie, eat your broccoli."

"Ah, Mom. Do I have to?" Then quietly to himself, "When I grow up and become President, I won't have to eat it any more."

And indeed, when little Georgie Bush became the 41st President of the United States, he banned broccoli from the White House.

Is this a wise decision on the part of President Bush, or is it an error in judgement?

The merits of broccoli, other green and yellow vegetables, fruits and vitamin A are being studied intensely, particularly because they *may* have a protective affect against certain cancers.

The term "vitamin A" is confusing because it includes both retinol, which is the dietary source of vitamin A from animal sources, and beta-carotene, the provitamin present in vegetables. The beta-carotene is ingested, stored as carotene and changed to retinol as needed.

The original interest in vitamin A occurred because of the diseases caused by its deficiency, usually in the diets of the poor. It is estimated that 16% of children's deaths in "developing countries" are due to the lack of this vitamin, which results in a reduction in the immune system and the loss of the ability to fight infections. Dryness of the skin, night blindness and total blindness can also be caused by a lack of vitamin A. Deficiencies are rare in the U.S. since the daily requirement of 3,000 IU (International Units) can be met by eating one stalk of broccoli, one bite of a carrot, or drinking several glasses of milk.

In experimental animals, vitamin A deficiencies were shown to cause pre-cancerous changes in the lungs and other organs. The exciting news is that some studies show that beta-carotene (the vitamin A in vegetables) may have a strong protective effect against lung cancer! A study of 2,107 men over a 19 year period revealed that the risk of developing lung cancer for long time smokers was reduced from 7% to 1% by doubling the amount of carotene (vegetable vitamin A) ingested. Unfortunately, this beneficial protection was not found with other types of cancers.

Several large investigations are being conducted around the world in order to determine whether or not beta-carotene, taken on a regular basis, would be prophylactic against cancer. Two Maui doctors and I are presently participating in the Harvard Physicians' Health Study. Along with 22,000 other male physicians, we take a red capsule every other day. The capsule may contain 50 mg of beta-carotene or it may contain sugar (a placebo). The study started in 1983 and should be completed in another three years, at which time we will learn whether or not those physicians taking the beta-carotene developed fewer cancers (all other factors being equal) than did those taking the sugar-pill. I will let my readers know as soon as I have been notified.

A diet rich in beta-carotene is probably beneficial, but one high in retinol (the pure vitamin A) may be dangerous to your health! Retinol, which is found only in egg yolk and liver, is stored in a person's liver after ingestion. In excessive amounts, retinol can cause increased pressure in the brain and swelling of the nerves to the eyes. However, to reach those toxic levels it is necessary to eat beef liver once or twice a week or a single meal of polar bear liver (18,000 IU of retinol/gm)—not a very likely diet for most people!

Beta-carotene, on the other hand, is not stored in a person's liver but in the fat beneath the skin. As the beta-carotene content increases in the fat, the skin takes on a yellow color. The individual may worry about having jaundice from hepatitis or a tumor. On questioning, he/she will admit to eating several carrots every day or having a papaya each morning. One carrot has 20,000 IU and one cup of papaya has 2,819 IU of carotene. Fortunately, the yellow clears by reducing the amount of carrots or papaya eaten and no harm is done. A stalk of broccoli contains 3,000 IU and I am unaware of anyone turning either yellow or green from eating too many.

Broccoli, carrots and other green and yellow vegetables are very important sources of beta-carotene which has been shown to be important to your health. President Bush's wife, Barbara, made light of his dislike for broccoli by saying, "Anyone who likes to eat fried pork rinds, can't be all good." I'm not sure I even want to know what "fried pork rinds" are.

FITNESS VS. MORTALITY

How would you like to decrease your chances of dying from a heart attack or cancer by at least 75% during the next eight years? Does this sound too good to be true? Not according to the Institute for Aerobics Research of Dallas, Texas, as reported in *The Journal of the American Medical Association* (11-3-89). Because of its important findings, the article was reviewed by all the national television networks and by *Time* magazine.

The study included 10,224 men and 3,120 women who received medical examinations at the Cooper Clinic in Dallas, Texas, from 1970 to 1981. Their physical fitness was measured by having them run on a treadmill, after which they were classified into levels 1 to 5 (1 being a couch potato and 5 being a marathon runner). The authors then combined levels 2 with 3 and 4 with 5 because of similar findings in these groups. Excluded from the study were any individuals who had diabetes, abnormal EKG's (the reading of the heart), or a history of heart disease or strokes. Thus, the study started with relatively healthy people. During the next eight years, 283 of the participants died, 73 from cardiovascular disease (such as heart attacks), 82 from cancer, and the others from accidents and other causes. When the fitness levels of the people who died were compared to the fitness levels of the survivors, the findings were amazing!

Among the men there were 66 deaths (27.5% of the total deaths) from cardiovascular causes (heart attacks, etc.). The rate of these deaths in the couch potato men (fitness level 1) was 24.6 per 10,000 person-years, while in the 4-5 level group it was only 3.1 per 10,000 person-years. **These statistics mean a decrease of 87% in the risk of dying from cardiovascular disease if you exercise regularly!**

There were only seven deaths from heart attacks or other cardiovascular causes among the 3,120 women. The age-adjusted death rates per 10,000 person-years fell from 7.4 for fitness level 1, to 0.8 for fitness levels 4-5. **Again there was a decrease—this**

time of 89%!

It is understood by most people that exercising is beneficial to the heart, but the study also showed that there was a lesser chance of dying from cancer when they remained physically fit.

The death rate for men from cancer declined 76% once they got off the couch and started daily exercise. The statistics were even more startling for women, showing a decrease of 93% between the women in fitness group 1 and fitness group 4-5! Although the authors of the article do not give a reason for this wonderful finding, it has been shown by other studies that regular exercise improves a person's immune system. Anyone who exercises regularly will agree that not only do they feel better, but they have fewer colds.

Another important discovery was that moderate daily exercise tends to eliminate or reduce the risks of dying from elevated cholesterol, elevated blood pressure, obesity, or heart attacks which occur as a family trait. However, the lowest death rates still occurred in the groups where these other risks were controlled and the person exercised. The only risk factor that could not be significantly reduced by exercising was smoking. Even marathon runners who smoked had a higher risk of dying from cancer or a heart attack than did the laziest of couch potatoes who didn't smoke.

One of the most interesting findings of the study was that the greatest benefits were found between the fitness levels 1 and 2-3. This means that a person can gain most of the benefits with daily *moderate* exercise, which does not include running a marathon. The authors of the study believe that a brisk walk of 30 to 60 minutes each day is sufficient to reach the 2-3 fitness category. They did not comment on other methods of exercising, but bicycling, rowing, and cross-country skiing machines will all help a person reach his/her "ideal pulse rate" and gain maximum cardiac benefit. (The target pulse rate is 70 to 85% of 220 minus the person's age. Therefore a 60 year old man should try to obtain a pulse rate of between 112 and 136 during his exercises).

People frequently ask, "Does exercising after the age of

sixty offer any protection from heart attacks?" The Dallas study answers this with a loud, resounding YES. The greatest decline in death rates, with an increasing fitness level, was among men 50, 60 and older! A good example is my friend, Dr. A. Y. Wong. Every morning he takes a brisk 45 minute walk, followed by breakfast at home and then work at the hospital where he assists in surgery. Dr. Wong is 72 years old and feels better with each passing year!

Before you start an exercise program, have a checkup by your physician. Ask him about the Dallas article in JAMA. If he hasn't read it yet, share with him the information you learned. Maybe he will join you for that morning walk, if he hasn't started already.

WALKING AND LIVING LONGER

Last week I had the pleasure of speaking to a local chapter of the AARP (American Association of Retired Persons). The healthy, active members confirmed the information I was about to give in my talk. Of the 25 members present, 17 were 70 years of age or older. I asked, "How many of you, who are 70 or older, presently smoke?" No one raised a hand. Then I questioned, "How many of you had smoked at least one pack of cigarettes a day for 40 or more years?" Only one of the 17 raised her hand, and she had quit many years ago. I then asked, "How many of you exercise regularly at least three times a week." All 17 proudly raised their hands. The 17 members who were 70 years of age or older, still healthy and active, had confirmed the secrets of living a long and healthy life: Don't smoke, and exercise on a regular basis!

The dangers of smoking become more evident with each passing year. It was recently reported that smokers will shorten their lives by 15 YEARS! This does not even address the increase in illnesses during most of their lives. Smoking even wipes out the benefits of regular exercising. I cannot emphasize too often that the single, most important health habit a person can have is **NOT TO SMOKE**. If you are young, **DON'T START**. If you are older and smoke, **STOP**.

How long will our bodies last if we take care them? There is more and more evidence that the human body should last 110 to 115 years, barring accidents, cancer and tidal waves. Some believe that **THE BODY DOESN'T WEAR OUT. IT "RUSTS" OUT FROM DISUSE!**

Over the past 40 years, many studies have shown that regular exercise decreases the chances of heart attacks and other illnesses. In the 1950's, one of the earliest studies revealed that mailmen who carried their bags of mail and walked from house to house had one-half the rate of heart attacks as their fellow workers who sat behind a desk all day. Every investigation since then has confirmed the benefits of regular exercise. Last year, a report from Dallas showed that moderate, regular exercise decreased the deaths from cardiovascular disease by 87% and decreased cancer deaths by 75%!

There are many different types of exercises which benefit the heart. Swimming, jogging, bicycling, aerobic exercises, rowing machines, "stair-climbers," stationary bicycles, and cross-country skiing machines are all excellent ways of exercising your muscles and your heart. But the easiest, best, and most natural form of exercise for people over 60 is walking.

Our "advancing" civilization has made walking seem outdated. People get in their cars and drive two blocks to the store to buy a small bag of groceries. Children wait for the school bus rather than walk a mile to school. (My kids are tired of my stories of walking two miles through snow to get to school in Denver.)

Brisk walking for 60 minutes three to five times weekly is the amount necessary to produce cardiovascular conditioning and reduce the risk of a heart attack; however, other health benefits will be realized at the same time. Fitness walking reduces tension and anxiety states for several hours after the walk. There may be an increase in a person's beneficial cholesterol (HDL). Walking is believed to increase the mineral content in bone and to slow the development of osteoporosis. And most important, regular exercising, such as brisk walking, has been shown to slow down the aging process as measured by a person's oxygen consumption (how much oxygen the body can utilize).

Here are some hints for enjoying and getting the most benefits from walking.

1. If you have any heart problems, such as an irregular heartbeat, or if you are prone to fainting because of a heart condition, see your doctor for a checkup and get his/her advice before starting your walking, or any other exercise program.

2. Buy comfortable walking shoes. This will be your only expense, so don't skimp on them. Good shoes will prevent pains in your feet, legs and back.

3. Walk with your spouse or a friend. An exercise should

be as enjoyable as possible.

4. When you walk, take good strides and swing your arms to get the most muscular activity possible. Your heart won't beat faster unless there is an increased need for oxygen in your muscles.

5. Learn to take your pulse. If you can't find it, have the nurse at your doctor's office show you how.

6. Your cardiac goal (how fast your heart should beat) can be calculated by subtracting your age from 220 and taking 75% of that number. So if you are 60, your goal should be a pulse of 120, at 65, a pulse of 116, at 70, a pulse of 112, at 75, a pulse of 108, and at 100, a pulse of 90!   At 110, I would be happy to have any pulse at all.

7. Start with a short distance, perhaps around the block. Do this daily for the first week. Then increase the distance each week until you have reached your cardiac goal.

You *can* increase your life span! Remember, **SMOKING *AND* INACTIVITY ARE HAZARDOUS TO YOUR HEALTH.**

SEAT BELTS

The sickening screech of the skidding tires... the loud crash of metal hitting metal...the body flying forward and hitting the window...a beautiful face cut to pieces. Blood, broken bones and death. All so sudden, so permanent. Can it be prevented?

Deborah left the hospital after three days. Her only injuries were those of a very stiff neck and a bruised tummy. Her beautiful face was not scratched and she was ALIVE! She had been in a serious auto accident and had heard the "skidding tires and the metal hitting metal," but she had been wearing a seat belt and it saved her life. Pictures of her car show complete destruction, with the engine pushed into the front window. She is lucky to be alive, but most would say it was more than luck. It was her decision to use her seat belt that saved her life.

When Deborah was admitted to the hospital, she had bruises across her left shoulder and her lower abdomen from the impact of her body onto the belt. An air bag would have prevented even these injuries.

Deborah's bruises have healed but more serious injuries associated with the use of seat belts can occur. A broken clavicle (the front shoulder bone) occurs rarely. But if the driver had not been wearing the belt, he/she would have hit the steering wheel with such force that the heart or the aorta (the large artery leaving the heart) would have been injured. The portion of the belt across the lap can occasionally rupture the small intestine, liver, spleen or urinary bladder. But the patient can be treated and survive these injuries, whereas he/she would not have survived the mutilation that would have occurred if the belt had not been worn. The seat belt has never injured the uterus of a pregnant women but the lap belt should be positioned below the uterus and the shoulder portion above the uterus. The seat belt will save the life of the fetus (the unborn child) by saving the life of the mother.

Critics of seat belt laws say that there has not been the decrease in the number of traffic deaths that had been expected. However surveys show that only 30-50% of drivers are wearing their belts and that there HAS been a decrease in THEIR deaths.

Have you ever looked at the front windshield of a car after it has been towed in from an accident? I cringe when I see the broken glass in the shape of a star-burst. The glass is always broken outward as a result of the head and face being thrown forward. The blood, the pain, the disfigurement always follows.

Deborah, thank you for letting me tell your story. Let's hope that the readers will "buckle up" and perhaps we will have saved a life or two.

Yes, accidents will happen. Without a seat belt, you may never remember the screech of tires or the crash of the metal. With one, you have a fighting chance.

PAP TEST

Cervical and uterine cancer remain as great threats to a woman's life, but the danger has been reduced during the last 40 years by the use of the Pap test. What is the Pap test? How important is it? How often should it be done?

The Pap test was named after Dr. George Papanicolaou (1883-1962) who discovered that cancer cells from a cervical cancer could be found in vaginal secretions. By finding the cancer early, before it had spread, surgery could be performed to save a woman's life. This test is considered the greatest single breakthrough of the twentieth century in the fight against women's cancer of the cervix.

Cancer of the cervix does NOT start suddenly and spread rapidly to other tissues. It is believed that the normal cervix (Class I Pap slide) first develops abnormal changes called atypia (Class II). These changes then progress into dysplasia (Class III) which is still not a cancer. Dysplasia then progresses into carcinoma in situ (Class IV) and finally to invasive carcinoma (Class V).

Carcinoma in situ is a very superficial, not deadly cancer. The invasive carcinoma (class V), however, spreads to adjacent organs and ultimately takes a woman's life. Researchers believe that it may take eight or more years for carcinoma in situ of the cervix to finally develop into invasive carcinoma. It is this length of time that allows women to be cured, particularly if the cancer is found in its early stages of growth and the necessary surgery can be performed.

The Pap test is an excellent screening method for detecting abnormal changes in the cervix, but what is the next step? Modern gynecology requires that a woman then have a colposcopic exam. This is an examination of the cervix with a magnifying microscope, and can be performed in the office. The cervix is stained and abnormal areas are biopsied.

Considerable disagreement has developed as to how often a woman should have a Pap test. Since the test was introduced in

1942 the recommendation had been to have a Pap test on an annual basis. Recently the American Cancer Society pointed out that if it takes eight years for the cancer to develop, then considerable savings would occur with less frequent testing. Their recommendations are that all asymptomatic women age 20 and over, and those under 20 who are sexually active, have a Pap test annually for two negative examinations and then at least every three years until the age of 65.

The Pap test, along with breast examination and guaiac testing of the colon, remains an extremely important test in detecting a woman's cancer early so that it may be removed and cease to threaten her life.

OSTRICH SYNDROME

Webster's Dictionary defines the word "syndrome" as "a group of signs and symptoms that occur together and characterize a particular abnormality." I define the "ostrich syndrome" as that condition when people stick their heads in the sand and refuse to consider the truth about a medical problem.

The ostrich syndrome occurs in all walks of life, but it is particularly prevalent in medicine. Daily you will see people not wearing their seat belts because "It can't happen to me." Or you hear them say, "I don't need a will 'cause I'm not going to die for a long time." "Next year is plenty of time to quit smoking." "I don't have to worry about my taxes until April."

Denial, procrastination, avoidance, fear—there are many reasons why we don't do what we should, and we all are guilty at one time or another.

As a surgeon, time and time again I see women who do not examine their breasts because they are afraid of what they might find. Some will actually ask, "Why look for trouble?" Others express the fear that examining their breasts might actually cause a cancer. Of course this is ridiculous, but because of these fears, women are missing the chance of finding tumors early and saving their lives. Nothing but education will change these attitudes. The American Cancer Society has spent millions of dollars over the past 50 years in order to correct these misconceptions and offer women a chance of beating this disease.

"I feel too well to be sick." "Don't fix it if ain't broke." "Everyone dies sometime." These are some of the rationalizations from men who avoid a physical exam. Annual physical exams for those who are between 20 and 40 may be a waste of money and of the doctor's time; however an exam at 40, 50 and annually thereafter is a wise investment in your future.

The most tragic example of the ostrich syndrome occurs when a young man or woman watches a black skin mole grow, and is afraid to see a doctor because it "may be a cancer." If it is a melanoma (a black skin cancer), a delay of only a few months can mean the chance of being cured decreasing from 99% to less than 50%!

A chronic cough in a smoker, rectal bleeding, vaginal bleeding, an enlarging lump under the skin, are all signs which say, "Get your head out of the sand and see your doctor."

There is good news! *The World Book Encyclopedia* assures us that ostriches *do not* stick their heads in the sand to avoid danger, although it is a commonly held belief. Therefore, there *is* no place to hide – for the ostrich or for us! See your doctor. Find out why you are coughing. Have him examine that mole. Ask him to teach you how to do a breast self-examination. Your good health depends on YOU. Don't be an ostrich.

OAT BRAN VS. WHEAT BRAN

"Tastes great!" "Less filling!" "Tastes great!" "Less filling!" We have all seen the TV beer commercials where the burly men are arguing about the qualities of a particular beer. Now imagine a scene in a health food store where two customers are arguing about the best type of bran. "Oat bran!" "Wheat bran!" "Oat bran!" "Wheat bran!" Who is right about the better bran? Both are, although oat bran is getting the most publicity today.

Bran is the outside coating of the grain, whether it be oats, wheat, rice or any other grain. As people became "civilized" they developed machines to "chew off" the outside coating, which was then discarded, so that the tender, soft inner part of the grain could be made into flour and other products. When the outside coating (the bran) was thrown away, civilized society set itself up for a whole pack of illnesses.

Bran and other types of vegetable fiber can be classified either as a soluble fiber (which can be dissolved in water) or an insoluble fiber (which cannot). It is this quality of solubility which gives each type of bran its special value. When the bran is insoluble, as with wheat bran, it remains in the intestinal tract and absorbs water to soften and add bulk to the stool. This results in the stool moving rapidly through the bowel and being expelled.

Soluble bran, such as oats and rice, is digested and absorbed into the body where it attaches to, and removes, bile. As the bile contains cholesterol, the cholesterol level in the blood will tend to decrease as more bile is removed. Soluble bran is also reported to help diabetic patients control their blood sugar levels, although the reason for this beneficial effect is not known.

Some medical researchers would have you believe that when civilization developed a taste for processed grain, and threw away the bran, the ills of the world descended on us. Heart disease, colon cancer, diverticulitis, appendicitis, breast cancer, prostate cancer, obesity, diabetes, gallstones, hemorrhoids, and varicose veins have all been blamed on the lack of fiber.

For the last 20 years, Dr. Dennis P. Burkitt has investigated the problems which can develop in the human body when there is a lack of fiber in the diet. His studies were based mostly on the investigation of African tribes that consumed high amounts of fiber, compared with the British and other populations that had small amounts of fiber in their diets. Many assumptions were made, and they are being born out in additional studies today.

Heart attacks were rare among the Africans and this fact was thought to be the result of a high fiber diet. More recent studies have shown that the soluble fiber absorbs the cholesterol and fats while the insoluble fiber allows it to be excreted more rapidly. These two properties will lower the cholesterol level in a person and reduce the risks of having a heart attack.

Colon cancer is extremely rare in societies with high fiber intake. The insoluble fiber, as in wheat, makes the food move quickly through the bowel so that the carcinogens (the chemicals which may cause a cancer) do not have time to act on the bowel wall. This same increase in the bowel motility and elimination of toxins (poisons) has been thought to decrease the chances of breast and prostate cancer.

A study of school age children in Seattle revealed a 50% decrease in the rate of appendicitis when the children had a whole grain diet.

What kind? How much? How often? How? These questions about bran need answering now that we know that it is important.

Since wheat bran doesn't absorb cholesterol and oat bran isn't as effective in softening the stool and decreasing transit time, it is obvious that **WE NEED BOTH WHEAT BRAN AND OAT BRAN IN OUR DIETS.**

How much, and how often? Researchers believe that three tablespoons of a mixture of wheat and oat bran will satisfy the daily needs for soluble and insoluble fiber. **DO NOT** try introducing bran into your diet with three tablespoonfuls all at once, you will experience considerable abdominal gas and discomfort. Start with **one teaspoon** of bran daily, and if you have no problems then increase it to two a day. Slowly, over three to four months, increase the amount of bran until you are taking **three table-spoonfuls** daily in different foods.

How? There are many recipe books on ways to use wheat and oat bran. You probably would not want to eat the bran by itself. It is quite "grainy" and sticks to your mouth. Adding a tablespoon of bran to your breakfast cereal is easy enough. "Breakfast cookies" are a tasty way to get your kids started on a healthy bran habit. Muffins, coffee cakes, waffles, pancakes, are other foods to which bran can be added. The list is endless: casseroles, breads, spaghetti, pasta, burritos, noodles, chicken, turkey, etc. . . .

Some "bran prophets" will guarantee that your stools will be soft and regular. Most likely you will lose some weight because you will not be as hungry and the foods will be carried quickly through the body. It *is* believed that you will have a lower risk of colon cancer and of heart attacks. Considering all the benefits of bran, why don't you start adding it to your family's meals.

BENEFITS OF WATER

My mother would harp at me to drink more water every day. As a typical boy, I would pour my glass of water into the sink when she wasn't watching. Now, 50 years later, I have learned that she was right. My sons now pour their glasses of water into the sink when I'm not watching.

What are the benefits of drinking water? How is water controlled in our bodies? Can you drink too much water?

The body is worth only a few dollars because 60% is water. The mechanisms which control that 60% are very elaborate and involve the hypothalamus (one of the areas of the brain), the pituitary gland (a gland at the base of the brain), the kidneys, and the adrenal glands.

When sweating, diarrhea or other fluid losses occur, the increased osmotic pressure (thickness) of the blood plasma stimulates the hypothalamus (the brain center) to produce the sensation of thirst. The person then drinks liquids in order to re-establish the body's normal state. The hypothalamus also stimulates the pituitary gland to release a hormone called vasopressin that circulates through the blood. When vasopressin reaches the kidneys, it turns down "the faucets," decreases the urine produced, and saves more water.

This process would seem to be enough of a control to regulate the body's water, but there is another important control mechanism. Sodium, part of the salt that we eat every day, is the most important ion (a charged molecule) circulating in our blood stream. The sodium and chloride ions hold onto water. A high level of sodium will produce a swollen plasma volume, which produces hypertension (high blood pressure). It also causes a swollen interstitial space (a space between the blood vessels and the body's cells) which appears as edema, such as swelling of the legs and feet. Therefore, a careful control of the sodium ion is necessary, and the body's adrenal glands perform this function.

When a person's diet is low in sodium, the adrenal gland secretes a hormone called aldosterone that causes the kidneys to save the sodium ion in the normal process of making urine. Likewise, in a healthy person with a diet of too much salt, the adrenal gland produces less aldosterone and the kidneys excrete more sodium in the urine. The body is a wonderful machine!

The kidneys are magnificent organs and life without them is extremely difficult and expensive. Each kidney is made up of over a million microscopic tubes called nephrons. Each nephron has a head, called a glomerulus, which in turn is attached to a long tubule (a microscopic tube). Approximately 25% of the body's total blood passes through the kidneys each minute. The glomeruli filter about 180 liters per day, but the tubules will reabsorb 99%, leaving a urine output of one liter per day. It is this ability of the kidneys to reabsorb the 179 liters that controls the body's water and sodium balances.

The kidneys not only control the body's water, but they also secrete, or remove, toxic waste products such as urea. Urea is the final waste product of the body's utilization of amino acids. It must be excreted by the kidneys or, as it builds up in the body's blood, confusion, coma and death will occur.

So what should you expect if you do not drink a normal amount of water? First, there will be an increased sensation of thirst and a decreased amount of urine produced as the body tries to compensate. The urine becomes more concentrated as the kidneys continue to do their work. With a more concentrated urine there is an increased risk of kidney stones.

As the dehydration continues, the body loses its ability to sweat and becomes susceptible to heat stroke. With a loss of body water, the plasma volume decreases and the individual notices increasing weakness. Water is also lost from the body's cells and poor skin tone is evident. Hopefully, the person will find some water and drink it before the final events of stupor, coma and death occur.

Water, the gift from heaven, is to be drunk and enjoyed. The benefits are significant and will improve your health. By increasing the amount of water consumed, the risk of kidney stones drops considerably. This fact was demonstrated by a study in two villages in Israel. The people in one village continued their normal consumption of water, while people in the second village increased their consumption so that the they would each be producing about 300 cc's (one cup) more of urine per day than was usual. Within three years, the incidence of kidney stones among people from the second village had fallen by 90%!

There are several other values of water. With a larger volume of fluid passing through the kidneys, more body toxins, such as urea, are removed and the individual will feel better. In addition, constipation will definitely decrease. The extra fiber that we eat in our diets cannot work if water is not available. The fiber binds onto the water and increases the bulk and softens the stool. Skin tone also improves. When our family travels to Colorado to ski, we all must drink four to six extra glasses of water a day to keep our skin and lips from drying out in the high, dry climate.

Most weight reduction programs encourage participants to drink two or three liters of water per day. I'm not sure that this actually helps a person lose weight, but it certainly removes all the waste products from the breakdown of the fat.

How much water should you drink a day in order to gain these benefits? Most physicians, myself included, recommend that you set a goal of drinking two liters (about two quarts) of water a day. That's 8 eight-ounce glasses! I'll admit that I have a hard time reaching that goal.

Alcohol and coffee will not work as substitutes because they arc both dehydrating. Ask someone who has had too much to drink the night before about how his mouth feels the next morning.

Don't worry about drinking too much water—as long as you are not eating excess salt at the same time. The normal kidneys can excrete 15-20 liters (almost five gallons) of urine a day! The body's regulatory mechanisms will do the rest.

For persons who are not trying to drink more water but still find themselves always thirsty and having to urinate frequently, I would recommend that they see a doctor immediately. These may be the signs of early diabetes and urgent treatment is needed.

There are some drawbacks from drinking eight glasses of

water a day. A long automobile trip will require several stops. Even I have been "inconvenienced" during a long operation after drinking my goal of water.

BREAST SELF-EXAMINATION

I continue to be alarmed by how few women examine their breasts for lumps on a regular basis. I ask every woman referred to my office for a breast examination, "How often do you examine yourself?" Fifty percent never examine themselves; twenty-five percent say, "Now and then," and only twenty-five percent reply, "Monthly."

As ninety percent of breast cancers are found first by the patient, it is extremely important that women practice breast self-examination to find any lumps as early as possible. How tragic it is when a patient tells her physician the story that "she bumped her breast and found a lump the size of an orange." Science knows that her cancer had been present for months and probably had already spread to other areas of her body.

Women who are afflicted with breast cancer *can* discover it early enough and improve their chances of survival. Here is how.

Mammograms are presently the best method of discovering a breast cancer at its smallest size, but mammograms miss 15 percent of cancers! Because few women obtain the rather expensive ($75-$100) mammogram every year, the most frequent, and cheapest, method of finding a breast cancer is a regular, careful examination by the patient. The American Cancer Society has called this BSE, Breast Self-Examination. Instructional booklets are available, but a refresher course is always beneficial.

First, take time to do it right. Don't rush—your life may depend on it. Stand in front of a mirror and place your hands on your hips. Press your hands down and look carefully at the skin on the breasts. If dimpling occurs in an area, then note and report it to your physician. This could be a sign of an underlying cancer.

Next, while still standing, gently "squeeze" the left breast between the fingers of the right hand. Gently "roll" the breast tissue while you feel with the finger tips. Feel for any lumps that are not similar to lumps in the rest of the breast. A hard lump the size of a pea may be a very important finding, particularly if it had not been felt during a previous exam. After you have examined the left breast, then examine the right breast with the left fingers. Occasionally lumps can be found in this manner that cannot be felt lying on your back.

The most important part of the exam is when the patient examines herself while lying on her back, with one arm raised over her head. This position tightens the breast tissue against the chest wall and makes it easier to find even smaller lumps. To examine the left breast, use the fingers of the right hand. Use the soft padded ends of the 2nd, 3rd and 4th fingers and, with a light, rolling motion, pretend that you are feeling for a pea inside a small soft pillow. Start at the top of the breast (12 o'clock) and in small rolling circles, proceed around the breast as though you were going around a clock. Go around once with light pressure and then again with firmer pressure. Be sure to examine in the arm pit while you are checking the breast. Lumps found in this area may signal trouble in the breast. When you have finished examining the left breast, then switch arms to check the right breast. Raise the right arm over the head while you examine the breast with the 2nd, 3rd and 4th fingers of the left hand.

"Doctor, my breasts are filled with lumps!" This is the cry of despair that causes many women to abandon examining their breasts. Ninety percent of women will have from one to a hundred lumps in their breasts. How can you tell which are benign and which threaten your life? If you have faithfully been checking your breasts, you will know what is "normal" for you and be able to identify any new or changed lumps. Otherwise you should see your physician in order to determine for the first time what is "normal" for you and what is abnormal. After that visit, it is up to you to remain familiar with the nodules or lumps in your breast in case any of them change or a new one appears. Once you find any abnormalities see your doctor!

How often should you examine your breasts? Is once every month or two often enough? No! I recommend that a woman check herself weekly to remember what the lumps in her breasts feel like. Who can remember from month to month the road maps of her breasts? In fact, it's a sad story that it's easier for women to forget the exam each month rather than remember to do it.

"But once a week is using 5-10 minutes when I could be . . ." You brush your teeth twice a day. How many women die from toothaches every year? FORTY-TWO THOUSAND women in the U.S. die each year from breast cancer. Many would have lived if their cancers had been found earlier.

Your chance of developing breast cancer is one in ten. Whether you die from it or recover may depend upon whether you discover it during one of your self-examinations. What are you waiting for?

3 Symptoms

PAIN

Oh! PAIN!

As a surgeon I am used to pain—other people's pain. But last week I had a toothache which drove me to my knees. It was a loose crown which was bouncing on a nerve root. Although I chewed on the "right side" of my mouth, if I bumped the left lower molar, I went to my knees with pain which would last 60 seconds (about a lifetime).

My dentist saw me the next day at noon, made a temporary repair and wanted to do the final repair on Friday. Because I had surgery scheduled on Friday, I made an appointment for the following week—the worst mistake of my life. No sooner had the dentist's office closed Friday afternoon than the crown came loose again. I was destined to eat mush over the weekend! Even when I ate soft foods, I would occasionally bump the molar and the pain would sear the left side of my face and extend up into the ear. It made a great diet plan as I developed an aversion to eating.

The nights were worse. I apparently "grind" my teeth when I sleep. I would be sound asleep and suddenly bolt upright with an excruciating pain in my jaw. After the pain abated, I would fall back to sleep only to jolt awake again an hour later. The nights were endless. Relief finally came on Monday, after the final repair had been completed.

Pain is a very important sensation for all of us. The survival of our bodies depends on it. (I would have denied this last weekend.) Without pain sensation, we would not drop the hot pan, and would step on the hot coals. We would be unaware that we were developing appendicitis or an ulcer. We would try to walk on a broken leg and be unaware that we were having a heart attack. Like it or not, pain helps us survive.

Almost all tissues and organs in the body have pain nerves connecting them with the brain, usually through complicated pathways. However, the nerves from the arms and legs also connect with motor nerves in the spinal cord. When you touch something hot, the impulse traveling to the brain will stimulate the motor fibers in the spinal cord and will cause you to withdraw your hand, even before the brain knows that you have been burned!

The pain nerves are made of two types of fibers, fast and slow. The fast fibers carry the pain impulse at 12 to 30 meters per second while the slow fibers at only 0.5 to 2 meters per second. This explains why you feel sharp pain suddenly (the impulses of the fast fibers) and then the lingering, aching pain (the impulses of the slow fibers). A tooth must be loaded with slow fibers!

Superficial pain can be localized so you will know exactly what is hurting. However deep pain is more difficult to localize and is what we experience with abdominal pain, chest pain or headaches.

Referred pain is interesting, in that the location of what is causing the pain is not where you feel it. Pain from a heart attack can be felt in the left arm and the pain from a ruptured spleen can be felt in the left shoulder. Although the appendix is located in the lower, right side of the abdomen, the discomfort from appendicitis is first noticed in the upper part of the abdomen.

My toothache has had a beneficial effect: I am more sensitive and sympathetic with my patients and their complaints about pain.

FEVER

You have a fever? Take two aspirin? Maybe not. One of the amazing parts of the ongoing study of medicine is that many beliefs which we hold very dear to us, as though they were written in stone, are questioned and even proved wrong as the years go by. Such is the case of treating slight fevers with aspirin or Tylenol.

Hippocrates, in his time, speculated that fever "cooked out excessive body humors," which he blamed for disease. Today we are starting to believe that he may have been correct.

For several centuries physicians treated their patients who had syphilis by infecting them with malaria and producing high fevers. The treatment may have been worse than the disease as the patient could die from either one.

Interestingly, cold-blooded vertebrates such as lizards and fish will seek out warmer environments when they are sick. Humans are also believed to be helped by low-grade fevers. When a bacteria or virus sets up an infection in the body, the white blood cells release a hormone called Interleukin-1, which stimulates the body to generate more heat by burning body fat and causing the muscles to shiver. The Interleukin-1 enhances immunity by also increasing an important white blood cell, called the T-cell, and the high temperature itself increases the activity of the body's natural virus-fighting substance, Interferon.

However, excessive body temperatures *can* be dangerous. In children, temperatures of 104 degrees or higher frequently cause convulsions. In adults, heat stroke may occur and be fatal. Moderate fevers of 100 to 102 should be treated with respect, and the patient should seek the advice of a doctor. Dr. Atkins of Yale advises that "if the cause is bacterial, antibiotics are usually the proper treatment. If it is viral, it may be wise to postpone the aspirin and give the fever a chance to do its ancient work."

I certainly believe that the body is a marvelous creation which has remarkable abilities to heal itself if it is cared for properly. I would agree that moderate fevers are not dangerous and may be of benefit, but please don't wait too long to see your physician.

ANGINA

"There is a disorder of the breast marked with strong peculiar symptoms....Those, who are afflicted with it, are seized while they are walking and most particularly when they walk after eating, with a painful and most disagreeable sensation in the breast, which seems as if it would take their life away, if it were to increase or to continue; the moment they stand still all this uneasiness advantages." This description of angina (or heart pain) is as true today as when it was written in 1772, by Dr. William Heberden.

The cause of this anginal pain is a narrowing of the coronary (heart) arteries from arteriosclerosis and an increased demand for oxygen to the heart muscle. When an individual is exercising, walking, under stress or has just eaten a large meal, the myocardium (heart muscle) needs more oxygen. If the arteries to the muscle have been narrowed by cholesterol deposits or by spasm of the artery, then an insufficient amount of oxygen reaches the muscle and Mother Nature warns us by producing pain. This causes us to stop what we are doing, and the pain disappears.

Angina is most often described as a tightness around the chest or a squeezing sensation. Sometimes it is just a "heavy chest" feeling. Frequently the discomfort will travel up to the jaw or to the left shoulder or left arm. With rest, the pain disappears within ten minutes. If the pain or discomfort remains, it means that the heart muscle continues to receive inadequate oxygen and that a heart attack may be occurring. Other conditions can cause similar pain: ulcers, a hiatal hernia or gallbladder disease. Because angina and a heart attack are the most dangerous, they MUST be investigated first.

Evaluation of the pain by your physician or a cardiologist (a heart specialist) will include a complete physical examination, an ECG (an electrocardiogram, or electrical reading of your heart) and, most likely, a treadmill stress test. This last test is very important because it frequently demonstrates a patient's physical condition. During the treadmill stress test, the patient is wired to an ECG so that the heartbeat and heart waves can be monitored every second. The patient starts to walk on the treadmill (a moving belt on a platform), and after a few minutes the speed of the belt is increased so that the patient must start to jog. Then the platform is tilted upward to simulate jogging uphill. The test continues as long as the patient is able to keep up with the treadmill or until abnormal changes are noted on the ECG. This test is extremely valuable and will usually detect the narrowing of the coronary arteries producing the anginal pain. I also recommend this "stress test" for men and women over the age of 40 who come from families where other members have had heart attacks. The test will frequently pick up narrowing of the arteries *before* a heart attack occurs.

If the "stress test" is abnormal, a cardiac catheterization may be ordered by the cardiologist. This is an x-ray of the arteries of the heart which clearly shows the degree of narrowing of the arteries. With this information, the physician can recommend several methods of treatment for the anginal pain.

The first mode of treatment, unless severe narrowing of the arteries has been determined by x-rays, is the use of drugs. Nitroglycerin tablets, placed beneath the tongue, have been used for over a hundred years, and are still as effective as ever in dilating the arteries in the heart. Skin patches of nitroglycerin are now used for a longer, more sustained dose; however, the body becomes adapted to prolonged use and the patches must be removed from time to time. Other cardiac (heart) medications used to treat angina include Procardia, Verapamil, Cardizem and Inderal.

If the angina is not controlled with the use of drugs, or if a severe narrowing of the arteries is found on the x-rays, then a direct attack on the arteries is necessary. If only one area of narrowing is found, then usually a balloon angioplasty is recommended. During this procedure a small tube is passed from an artery in the leg up to the narrowed artery in the heart. A small balloon on the end of the tube is inflated in the narrowed segment, and the cholesterol plaque is squeezed to the side. In this manner the narrowed segment is reopened, more blood can reach the heart muscle, and the angina should clear. The procedure is successful 90% of the time, but unfortunately 30% of the arteries will clog again within one year. Moreover, emergency surgery is required 5% to 10% of the time because of an injury to the artery during the procedure.

For the past 20 years the primary type of surgery for angina has been coronary artery bypass surgery. Veins taken from the legs are attached to the aorta (the large artery just above the heart) and then to the small arteries in the heart, bypassing the narrowed areas. In this manner, three, four, five, or more narrowed areas can be bypassed. With the excellent cardiac surgeons and teams today, the mortality (death rate) is only 1% to 3%, and 80% of the veins should still be working at the end of one year.

Laser surgery is still in the experimental stage, with the aim to "burn out" the cholesterol plug without burning a hole in the wall of the artery.

Although drugs, balloons and surgery are available to treat the pain of angina, why not take better care of your heart and avoid the need for these treatments? Control your cholesterol, stop smoking, exercise regularly and have an annual physical examination.

LEG CRAMPS

At one time or another we have all awakened at night with terrible cramps in the calves of our legs. None of us will forget the frantic massaging of the calf or pulling the toes back to try to gain relief from the severe pain. Nocturnal leg cramps are one of the many aches and pains which affect our legs. There are dozens of causes of leg cramps, but three of the more common ones are important to know about.

Exertional leg cramps can affect even the best trained athletes. These athletes, whether in high school, in college or professional, can find themselves falling to the ground and clutching their leg, and then out of play for the next five to ten minutes. The cause of this leg cramp is the loss of sodium and potassium from the muscle. They are lost through the great amounts of perspiration resulting from hard play during the game. Marathon runners try to prevent these cramps by replenishing their electrolytes with special drinks throughout their 26 mile race.

A completely different type of leg pain is intermittent claudication. This is a leg cramp that usually occurs in older individuals because of a lack of blood supply to the leg muscles. The arteries in the legs are simply pipes, and these pipes become clogged with arteriosclerosis (layers of cholesterol deposits) as the years go by. A narrowing is finally produced and the artery lets only enough oxygenated blood through to take care of the muscles while they are at rest. Leg cramps will occur after walking only short distances (one half block or less) because there is not enough oxygen getting to the muscles. After stopping for a few minutes, the leg cramps disappear but reappear with resumed exercise. If you have these symptoms, a vascular surgeon can "clean out" or replace these clogged pipes with new pipes, using other veins and/ or knitted Dacron tubes.

We all have painfully vivid memories about nocturnal leg cramps! Physicians do not really know why these cramps occur; however, electrical studies show frequent bursts of nerve stimuli which cause continual muscle contraction. Many different methods are used to treat nocturnal leg cramps, and most of them are successful. Quinine tablets taken before bed tend to relax the muscles and prevent the cramps. Other muscle relaxants are also successful.

The most natural method of reducing leg cramps is practiced by the long distance runner who stretches his leg muscles on a routine basis. One physician reported 44 patients who were relieved of nightly leg cramps through stretching exercises. He recommends standing three feet from a wall, and then leaning forward onto the wall leaving the heels on the floor. This stretches the calf muscles. Stretching for ten seconds, resting five seconds, and repeating this sequence three times is all it takes. All patients were reported cured of their cramps within one week and remained free of the leg cramps throughout the following year. Most of these individuals exercised intermittently after the first week.

Try the stretching method to reduce or eliminate nighttime leg cramps. But if you experience cramps in your legs after walking short distances, see your physician to be evaluated. Sweet dreams!

HOARSENESS

When a patient complains of hoarseness it is like waving a red warning flag to the physician. So when Bob came to my office complaining that his voice had been hoarse for the previous month, I immediately made an appointment for him to see Dr. Andrew Don, an otolaryngologist (ear nose and throat specialist). Bob was found to have a paralyzed vocal cord caused by a tumor in the lung. There are many causes for hoarseness, and fortunately most of them are not cancer! A knowledge of these causes could help you seek medical care at an appropriate time.

The production of the voice is a combination of air from the lungs passing over the vocal cords in the throat and then being "formed" by the tongue and lips. The vocal cords give the voice the resonance and pitch, while the tongue and lips articulate the air and turn it into words. If the vocal cords become swollen or thickened, then the voice falls in pitch. If the cords cannot come together the voice becomes breathy and weak. With this understanding, let us examine some conditions that cause a change in the voice.

Every boy who has gone through puberty has had his voice "change" by getting lower in pitch. The increased testosterone causes a permanent thickening of the vocal cords with the result being "the male voice." Myxedema, caused by an underactive thyroid gland, also causes thickening of the cords and a lower pitch in the voice. However, this is reversible with proper treatment.

The most common cause of hoarseness is laryngitis, or an infection of the "voice box" or vocal cords. This is frequently associated with a viral "cold" and subsides after several days of rest and medications.

Overuse of the voice can produce nodules on the vocal cords which are called "singer's or screamer's" nodes. The nodules change the vibration of the air as it passes over the vocal cord with a resulting raspy and breathy voice. Cheerleaders, salesmen, singers, ministers and politicians may develop them. The only treatment is resting the voice, something very hard for these individuals to do.

A paralysis of one of the vocal cords will cause a weak, breathy voice, since most of the air is lost with only one cord holding it back. The paralysis occurs after an injury to the nerve supplying the muscle within the cord. This may follow an operation on the thyroid gland, a viral infection or result from an invasion of the nerve by a cancer in the neck or chest.

The greatest concern of the physician about a patient's hoarseness is the possibility of a cancer on or near the vocal cords. Cancer of the larynx (the area around and including the vocal cords) accounts for only 1% of all malignancies, but in 1988 there were 12,000 cases in the United States and 3,800 deaths.

The causes are cigarette smoking and alcohol abuse, a deadly combination. It is believed that 95% of these patients could be cured if their disease was diagnosed at its earliest stage. The sad fact is that once diagnosed, only 63% of these patients live 5 years or longer because the cancer is usually too advanced. Earlier diagnosis by the patient or the doctor could increase the years of life.

If the cancer of the larynx starts on the vocal cord (it occurs there 80% of the time), a change in the voice can be noticed when the tumor is no larger than the size of a pin head. Mild hoarseness is the first sign. Breathiness, severe hoarseness, then increased effort in speaking are the advancing signs.

Early diagnosis of laryngeal cancer requires that the vocal cords and other areas of the larynx be examined carefully by a skilled physician. Most physicians learned to use an indirect laryngeal mirror in medical school and then quickly forgot it after graduation. The patient, therefore, is usually referred to an otolaryngologist for examination and treatment.

I cannot stress too strongly that a person over the age of 40, who has an episode of hoarseness lasting up to two weeks, should be seen by a physician for diagnosis, treatment and possible referral. The hoarseness following your cheering at the football game may be just a "screamer's node," but then again it could be something more serious.

HEADACHES

I have several patients who have migraine headaches from time to time. Recently, one remarked that a person who is experiencing a migraine should at the very least have blood coming out the eyes and ears so that the people around would know how badly it hurts. Perhaps then there would be more sympathy and an attempt at understanding the migraine patient.

Fortunately not all headaches are migraines; unfortunately a few are worse. Everyone will have a headache at one time or another, but only 5-10% will suffer from a migraine. About 80% of headaches are "tension" or psychogenic in origin and about 10-15% result from a variety of causes, such as an illness, a head injury, sinusitis, or a brain tumor, to mention a few.

Migraines are classified in a group termed "primary vascular headaches." Their cause and symptoms are believed to be due to the behavior of the blood vessels adjacent to the brain. They are considered hereditary, which is evidenced by my own experience: both my wife, her sister and our fourteen-year-old son suffer from them. An attack will usually be triggered by one of several factors and, unless the patient is able to stop the headache progression, a full blown migraine occurs which lasts from several hours to several days. Triggering dietary factors include alcohol, caffeine, and the food additives monosodium glutamate (MSG) and sodium nitrite. Environmental factors such as bright lights, strong odors and high altitude, certain drugs (vasodilators to treat hypertension and coronary artery disease), emotional factors, and estrogen changes in the female, are all guilty of starting a migraine. Even a small amount of the triggering factor, such as cooking fish with wine, may be enough to initiate a headache.

When the trigger is pulled, there is a shotgun blast of happenings with fancy medical terms like "platelet aggregation," "release of serotonin and thromboxane A2," "prostaglandins," "kinins" and "sterile arteritis." Essentially what happens first is a constriction or tightening of the blood vessels. The patient feels cold and clammy and knows that a migraine attack is on its way! Frequently an "aura" of sparkling lights will be seen. Soon the blood vessels adjacent to the brain dilate causing the severe, violent, pounding headaches. Abdominal cramps, vomiting and diarrhea follow, ensuring that the patient is thoroughly miserable. The attack will last several hours to several days and will leave the patient exhausted for the next 24 hours.

Is there any hope for migraine sufferers? Fortunately, yes. First they must avoid all triggering factors such as alcohol, caffeine, etc.... Next, if the attacks occur more than once a month then several drugs are available which block the chemical reactions that cause the arteries to dilate and produce the attack. Propranolol (Inderal) is the most effective and frequently used drug. It must be taken on a daily basis and will prevent most of the attacks. Propranolol must be avoided by people with asthma, myocardial insufficiency (a weakened heart muscle) and peripheral vascular disease (clogged arteries in the legs). Other medications which have been found effective include tricyclic antidepressants, calcium blockers, and antiserotonin agents.

The most common type of headache is the "muscle contraction headache" formerly known as the "stress" or "tension" headache. The patient usually complains of a steady, bandlike ache rather than the throbbing pain of a migraine. The pain is located at the back of the head or in the neck, whereas a migraine is most often felt in the front or side of the head. As the name implies, contraction or tightness of the neck and scalp muscles is present. Emotional factors, such as family or work related tensions, are usually to blame, but other causes may include arthritis of the neck, sinusitis, eye diseases and high blood pressure. Fortunately, controlling the blood pressure, treating the eye or sinus problem, or using some mild pain medication will control the acute attack. If the headaches are recurrent and due to emotional factors, then counseling, psychotherapy, mild tranquilizers or antidepressants are useful. In addition, biofeedback has been shown to offer definite benefits in preventing repeated attacks.

Headaches in children are worrisome because some have very

serious causes. Children can experience migraine and tension headaches as do adults, but less frequently. A headache in a child, who has not experienced them before, should be investigated immediately, especially if the child has a stiff neck, fever or a change in his degree of alertness. Recurrent headaches which increase in severity must also be investigated because they may indicate increasing pressure from a brain tumor.

Less common, but more serious, adult headaches include those resulting from a hemorrhage into the brain from a small vessel or from a "berry aneurysm." Occasionally, small blisters, called aneurysms, will form on the major blood vessels of the brain. When the blister starts to leak, a headache, usually severe, will occur as a warning signal. Once the aneurysm ruptures, a major stroke with paralysis or death will result. Early, delicate surgery may prevent this unfortunate outcome.

Another rare and serious headache in adults is associated with "temporal arteritis." The temporal artery lies in front of the ear and may become involved in an inflammatory process, causing the headaches. The headaches, however, are only a warning of an illness which may proceed to affect the arteries to the eyes and result in blindness. Early diagnosis and treatment with steroid medications can prevent this outcome.

Headaches developing even several weeks after an injury to the head should be evaluated by a physician. A blood clot, termed a subdural hematoma, resulting from the injury, may be expanding, causing the pain and threatening your life. Finally, the onset of severe headaches after the age of 35 may be the first sign of a brain tumor.

X-rays are of little assistance in diagnosing migraine or tension headaches. However, the CT or "CAT scan" is invaluable in detecting blood clots, a hemorrhage, or tumors of the brain.

Now that you have a thumbnail outline of the causes of headaches, the next time your spouse says, "Not tonight sweetheart. I have a headache," you can ask yourself, "Is it a migraine, or temporal arteritis, or, or?"

BACKACHES

I still vividly remember bending over and twisting as I reached for my dog, Max. The instant pain in my back was as though someone had stuck a knife deep into my spine. The next two weeks, as I lay in bed slowly recovering, I developed a great deal of sympathy for patients with back problems. "Your Aching Back" (*US News and World Report*, 10-17-84) by Dr. Augustus White, a professor of orthopedic surgery at Harvard Medical School, is an important contribution to understanding back problems and treatment, especially since 80% of all adults will have one sooner or later. (I'm still looking for the other 20%).

There are about 50 different causes of backaches, including wear and tear, arthritis, strains and sprains, minor and major injuries, pregnancy, and even illnesses, such as cancer located in other areas of the body. Men and women are affected about equally and the peak age is between 30 and 50.

Dr. White compares the parts of the spine to a stack of tin cans (the bony vertebrae) with jelly doughnuts (the discs) between them. As we get older the discs (or doughnuts) tend to dry out, the crusts weaken and tear (causing pain) and the center jelly may be squeezed out (a ruptured disc), resulting in pressure on a nerve and causing sciatic pain.

When asked about the best treatment for a backache, Dr. White replied, "Buffered aspirin, combined with bed rest, is still the best choice." The least expensive and safest treatment for a case of acute back pain is to lie down on your back with pillows under the knees and to take aspirin every 4 hours for 10 days to two weeks. If the pain persists after this conservative treatment then you should be evaluated by an orthopedic or neurosurgeon. A myelogram (an injection study of the spine) will be performed to look for the herniated (ruptured) disc. A CT scan will provide the same diagnostic information for those who wish to avoid the pain of an injection.

Surgery to remove the herniated disc (the jelly of the doughnut) may be necessary in order to relieve the pressure on the nerve.

Another procedure is to dissolve the jelly by injecting the disc with the enzyme called chymopapin. Success occurs in 75% of cases; nevertheless there have been rare, but fatal, side effects from the injection.

How can you prevent backaches and injuries to the disc? Exercises which strengthen the abdominal muscles and stretch the lower back are good. Swimming is excellent. In my own case, windsurfing has helped. Walking and bicycling are generally good, but golf, bowling, tennis, and baseball increase the risk of back trouble. When lifting, bend at the hips and knees, not at the waist. Lift with your leg muscles, not your back muscles. Sitting at a desk is bad for the back. If you have back trouble, use a "standing desk" when you read, type or write.

When asked, "Do people have back pain because they don't walk on all fours like animals?" Dr. White replied, "We know that animals who walk on all fours—dogs, for example—also have back pain. They just don't complain about it."

ABDOMINAL PAIN

From time to time everyone will have abdominal pains, and everyone, even physicians, begin to worry if they last more than a few minutes. Encircled by skin and muscles, the abdomen is a mysterious area containing many organs which are capable of having numerous problems. I would like to explain how a doctor categorizes his/her thinking in trying to determine the origin of the pain. There may be other signs or symptoms, such as fever, jaundice, or bleeding, but I am going to discuss only the symptom of pain in making a diagnosis.

For the last century, physicians have divided the abdomen into an upper area and lower area, and then subdivided each of these into three areas. Therefore, the patient has a right upper area (the right upper quadrant), the middle area (epigastrium) and the left upper area (the left upper quadrant). The lower half is divided into the right lower quadrant, the suprapubic area and the left lower quadrant. Granted, a quadrant is one-fourth of a circle and we now have six parts, but physicians are usually poor mathematicians. On the back, physicians refer to the right flank, the mid-back, and the left flank. Pain occurring in a particular area directs the physician's thinking along certain tracks toward making the diagnosis.

The severity of the pain determines the rejection or acceptance of a particular diagnosis. I classify pain as moderate, severe or catastrophic. Catastrophic pain is rarely localized but is usually felt throughout the abdomen. The causes of such pain would include a perforated (ruptured) ulcer, a ruptured aortic aneurysm (a blowout of the big artery in the abdomen), a ruptured diverticulitis or appendicitis with peritonitis (generalized infection), a ruptured ectopic (tubal) pregnancy in a woman, and abdominal trauma with injury to many organs.

In the right upper quadrant of the abdomen, moderate pain can be the result of a gallbladder attack, constipation, pneumonia, muscle strain, pyelonephritis (an infection of the kidney) or an enlarging liver (for one of many reasons). Severe pain in this area could be an infected gallbladder, diverticulitis of the colon in that area, and, rarely, appendicitis. Severe pain in the right flank is usually due to either a kidney stone or kidney infection, but a gallbladder attack can begin with pain in this area. Moderate pain in the epigastrium (the mid-upper abdomen) is present with ulcer disease of the stomach or duodenum, early appendicitis, hiatal hernia, and gallbladder disease. Severe pain in this area is felt when an ulcer begins to penetrate (ready to perforate), in pancreatitis (severe inflammation of the pancreas gland) and occasionally during a heart attack.

The left upper quadrant seems to have less trouble. Pains in this area are usually due to the colon (as with constipation or diverticulitis) or the spleen (when it enlarges, as with infectious mononucleosis).

Pain in the right lower quadrant of the abdomen is a real challenge for physicians, especially surgeons and gynecologists, as many problems can exist there. The first diagnosis that comes to mind is that of appendicitis, yet it is not the most common cause of right lower quadrant pain. Constipation probably leads the list. In children, mesenteric adenitis (swollen lymph glands) can mimic appendicitis. Kidney stones, tumors, diverticulitis of the colon, and inguinal hernias can cause pain in this area. In women, endometriosis, ovarian cysts and tumors, twisted fibroids, ectopic pregnancies, and infections in the fallopian tubes add to the challenge of diagnosis. (Now you can appreciate your physician's dilemma in making the correct diagnosis.)

The suprapubic area (mid-lower abdomen) is the area where the pain of cystitis (an infection in the urinary bladder) is noted. However, all of the female problems can be felt here.

Finally the left lower quadrant is the most frequent site for diverticulitis and its resulting pain. Again, ovarian cysts, ectopic pregnancies and infected fallopian tubes can cause pains here. In children, pain in this area usually occurs from constipation.

The pain from intestinal obstruction is not usually localized to one area, but is felt throughout the abdomen.

Books have been written on this subject and I apologize to my colleagues for omitting diagnoses such as internal hernias, herniated discs, ischemic bowel, and prostatitis. The correct diagnosis of abdominal pain may be difficult for even the expert, so please don't try to "diagnose yourself" to save a doctor's fee. See your personal physician as soon as possible and you might prevent a worsening of your condition.

GAS IN THE FAST LANE

After a patient has had surgery on the stomach, small intestine, or colon, doctors and nurses are always anxious for the patient to begin passing gas, as this is a sign that the intestine is once more working. Two years ago I had performed a major abdominal operation on Jack T.... After his recovery, he presented me with this article, "GAS IN THE FAST LANE". Using my "editing license," I am including this humorous anecdote in *TWO ASPIRIN – SECOND DOSE.*

....

Having never experienced the workings of the surgical ward in a hospital, I was totally unprepared for the importance of passing gas as a therapeutic process. As a first-time patient, it came as a social shock to be confronted, each meeting, by a group of strangers — nurses, nurses' aides, dieticians, blood pressurers and blood takers — with the greeting, "Have you passed gas today? Oh, good. A lot?"

My experience with passing gas began, as every male will remember, in about the third grade, when the boys in the back of the room would quietly and odorously try to outdo each other amid much nose holding, giggles and paper waving. From that beginning, gas passing grew into a competition between who could do it the loudest (junior high school), to who could do it the longest (high school), to who could do it most successfully and have it blamed on someone else (the mature ultimate).

So, as I was introduced to this new concept of passing gas as a means to start conversations, I was opened up to entirely new ways of looking at it. I began to think that here in the hospital, patients were somehow graded on how well they performed in the gaseous arena. Maybe, I thought, after each member of the team of specialists had completed his/her rounds, the team met to rank their patients. I didn't know what the rewards were, but it soon became obvious that it was going to be an advantage to be in the top third of the list. It was also obvious that this was a way to please the staff. With this thought in mind, I tried to prepare for visits by moving around a lot, drinking all my milk at each meal (because of its gas-producing qualities) and straining off a "posterior salute" whenever one of the team happened by. The professional staff was, however, prepared for patients' tricks and eagerness to please so they popped in at unscheduled times to put stethoscopes to abdomens and check out the rumblings. Through this method, they verified "passers" and quickly identified patients who were really not contributing. There was no hiding from these professionals.

These thoughts led me to believe that there may be some kind of award or reward given to the medical team member who was first in with a new gas report or who recorded the most successful performers or the most consistent or whatever. Maybe teams were competing for the best team total at the end of the week, with the winners earning an extra day's vacation or a free meal at Taco Hut. I know each new report was verified by another staff member. They would come in, pick up the chart at the foot of the bed and say, "Oh, you passed gas today."

Then I thought of the "gas pool" and realized this was probably the answer to staff boredom in the hospital. I envisioned, on a wall at the nurse's station, a row of numbers with new patients' names after each number. I guessed that staff members, for 25¢, drew a number representing a patient. The first new patient reporting a verified release, won for his number-holder whatever was in the pot that day; or maybe it was like an anchor pool where the time of the report is listed and the person who had drawn that time was the winner; or maybe it was the patient who went the longest without the blowing of the wind. I don't know the answers. I do know that this social phenomenon ends quickly once one leaves the confines of the medicated walls and returns to the world of the well.

Having been one of the hospital successes, I have found it difficult to attend social functions without "embarrassing moments."

....

Jack, thank you for your article. We all wish you luck with your "embarrassing moments."

4 Illnesses

GOUT

For the last thousand years, gout has been described as the disease of kings and the king of diseases. Imagine a picture of a medieval king with his swollen foot elevated on a pillow. Small demons are sticking pitchforks into his big toe, urging you to visualize how painful this disease can be and suggesting that it be blamed on the rich foods that kings consume. Apparently we have a thousand kings (and queens) on Maui, as gout is a common ailment in our island paradise.

Gout still presents itself most commonly as an extremely painful swelling and redness of the first toe, frequently following a minor injury. It can, however, affect the other joints making a diagnosis of gout, and not another arthritis, difficult.

Gout, and its accompanying pain, occurs when the uric acid in the blood crystalizes like small snowflakes and irritates or injures the joints. Uric acid is the product of "purine metabolism in man," or the breakdown by our body of the purines which are found in meat extracts, especially organs (such as pancreas, liver, and kidneys). As purines are not found in cereals and dairy products, a low purine diet is safe for a person with gout. Uric acid is not harmful in our blood stream until it rises above the level of 7mg% at which point crystals can form.

There are two usual circumstances when the uric acid level is elevated to 7mg% or over. The first condition is caused by either a diet of excess meats or a faulty metabolism of the body. The second condition is when the kidneys fail to excrete the normal amounts of uric acid.

How do physicians treat this extremely painful form of arthritis? The drug of choice when an acute attack occurs is colchicine, which can be given either by pill or by injection into a vein. Other drugs can be effective, such as Indocin, Butazolidin and Naprosyn. Regardless of their effectiveness in stopping acute attacks, doctors and patients must watch for possible negative side effects.

Once the acute attack has subsided (which can take several days), consideration should be given to lowering the uric acid level in the blood. A diet avoiding alcohol, meats and purine products is helpful, but patients rarely follow it. The drug allopurinol or Zyloprim is effective in lowering the serum uric acid if the body is over-producing. If the kidneys are not excreting as much uric acid as they should, then Benemid or Anturane are usually the drugs of choice.

I have always known that we have many kings and queens on Maui by the numbers who suffer from gout. One of our "jobs" as physicians is to dethrone the royalty.

SLEEP APNEA

Have you driven your wife from the bedroom with your snoring? Do you awaken with headaches and find that you are falling asleep during the day at work, or even while driving? You may have sleep apnea, but help is on the way.

Sleep apnea is a failure to breathe while sleeping. It can begin at any age and, if carried to the extreme, may be fatal. Usually, obese middle aged men are the victims of this strange affliction.

On an average, we take a breath once every five seconds while sleeping. Apnea is defined when the interval between breaths increases to greater than 10 seconds—and is often 15 to 60 seconds. With sleep apnea there must be at least 30 of these episodes during a seven hour sleep. It is not uncommon to have 300 to 500 of them if the illness is advanced.

If breathing is inadequate while we sleep, there are several important changes that occur in our bodies. The CO_2 (carbon dioxide) produced by the body is not removed and hypertension (high blood pressure) develops. The inadequate oxygen in the blood (hypoxemia) will cause sleepiness the next day, and may cause intellectual and personality changes if the illness is chronic. Slowing of the heart and irregular heartbeats are also common.

Three types of sleep apnea are recognized: obstructive apnea (the most common), in which the airway is blocked, central apnea, where the breathing impulse from the brain stops, and a mixed form combining both of these causes. The most common type of obstruction is from the tongue falling backwards and blocking the throat. Other problems of enlarged tonsils or adenoids, a deviated septum, an abnormal jaw or an enlarged tongue can cause an obstruction to the flow of air. Central apnea can be found in people with strokes, tumors at the base of the brain and poliomyelitis.

So, if you are snoring at night, sleepy the next day, have high blood pressure, and your wife tells you that your intellect and personality have hit bottom, how can you find out whether or not you have sleep apnea? You need the services of a sleep laboratory. While you sleep, a "polysomnogram" will be performed that measures your ECG (the reading of the heart), your EEG (the reading of the brain), the amount of air that you breathe, your breathing patterns, and the saturation of your blood with oxygen. With all this information the physicians will be able to tell whether or not you have sleep apnea.

Once sleep apnea is diagnosed, there is treatment. In patients with central apnea (where the brain is not telling the lungs to work) several drugs are used to stimulate the respiratory or breathing center of the brain. These include theophylline, progesterone (a female hormone), and acetazolamide. If these do not work, then breathing a low concentration of oxygen while sleeping will occasionally clear the problem.

Treating "obstructive" sleep apnea may be more difficult. Obese patients must first lose weight. Then drugs to stimulate the breathing can be tried. Breathing oxygen at night, in an attempt to increase the oxygen saturation of the blood, has produced both good and bad results. Another method, that of forcing air into the lungs with pressure and a tight fitting mask, has been beneficial. Surgery to remove the tonsils, adenoids and uvula has helped in 60% of cases. Finally, a tracheostomy (placing a breathing tube through the skin of the neck and into the trachea) gives 100% relief, but the long-term complications of this method may outweigh its benefits.

So, if you snore at night, fall asleep during the day, have high blood pressure and notice personality changes, see your doctor and ask whether sleep apnea may be the source of your problems.

CONSTIPATION

One of the most common conditions afflicting civilized man is constipation. No one escapes from an occasional attack, as when traveling. However some patients have chronic, almost incapacitating, constipation. What is it? Why does it occur? Is it ever dangerous? Are there any "home remedies?"

Constipation is defined differently by patients and doctors, but by and large, it is the failure to have at least three bowel movements a week. It is not limited to the later years of life; in fact it can be found among newborn infants when the nerves to the bowel fail to develop in a condition known as Hirschsprung's disease.

Epidemiologists tell us that constipation is a price we pay for civilization because most of the grains we eat have been "purified" and the fiber discarded. Indeed, constipation is unknown in Africa and other countries which are undeveloped and where people eat unpolished grains.

Constipation certainly is uncomfortable, and it can be dangerous. Sudden onset in middle or older ages could be the first sign of a cancer of the colon, and an examination by the family physician is indicated. Other illnesses such as diabetes, hypothyroidism (an underactive thyroid), diverticulosis, hernias, anal fissures, and hemorrhoids may also cause constipation. Certain medications, such as codeine in cough syrups, will slow the activity of the bowel resulting in infrequent movements.

One common cause of chronic constipation is the habitual use of laxatives. When a person relies on laxatives to "stimulate" the bowel, the colon becomes weaker in its own ability to achieve stimulation, and eventually is unable to perform without them.

After excluding these causes of constipation, the family physician will usually start the patient on dietary fiber for treatment. Most fiber comes from grain. (Vegetables and fruit contain a high water content and relatively little of the needed fiber). The greatest source of fiber is raw bran. Large amounts of bran may increase gaseousness and cause abdominal cramps. It is important to start with 1 teaspoonful of bran per day (probably with cereal) and gradually build to the necessary level which may be 1/3 to 1/2 a cup of bran a day mixed with different foods. It is also important to drink enough water, three to four glasses per day, so the bran will remain moist and soften the stool.

Another source of fiber is available from whole grain breads. A large bowl of granola every morning will also supply not only fiber but considerable protein.

Other "home remedies" are the use of Metamucil or Fiberall which contain psyllium mucilloid, a grain extract. This compound swells with water, adds soft bulk to the stool, and assists the colon in achieving a more natural movement.

Decreased physical activity may lead to constipation. This is especially true among nursing home patients or in many patients lying in bed after an operation. Walking can act as a laxative for older patients, and running is very effective for those who are younger and in good health.

One procedure, "high colonic irrigations" to relieve constipation, may be dangerous as both infections and deaths have been reported after their use. Avoid this solution to constipation in favor of other remedies.

"IT" is certainly an uncomfortable and bothersome problem but a thorough investigation by your physician to exclude the dangerous causes and then a proper diet and exercise program will correct most cases of constipation.

CHRONIC FATIGUE SYNDROME

"Yuppie flu" or Chronic Fatigue Syndrome—does it really exist or is it just an excuse for the "tired young?" According to the Centers for Disease Control (CDC) in Atlanta, Georgia, and a recent national meeting in San Francisco, a new illness known as the Chronic Fatigue Syndrome (CFS) does exist and deserves the attention and understanding of the medical profession.

The CDC requires that for a patient to be diagnosed as having this illness there must be persistent or relapsing, debilitating fatigue lasting at least six months. Other causes of such fatigue must be excluded, such as cancer, chronic inflammatory disease, chronic psychiatric disease, drug abuse, endocrine (glandular) diseases and others. The patient may also complain of mild fever, sore throat, painful lymph nodes or glands in the neck, headaches, joint pain (without swelling or redness), sleep disturbance, unexplained muscle weakness, and neuropsychologic complaints such as photophobia, confusion, irritability, inability to concentrate or depression.

Researchers have been unable to determine the cause, predict its course, or offer a cure. There are many doctors who doubt that it exists at all. Other physicians believe that it may be a form of chronic mononucleosis (a viral disease), or a chronic Epstein-Barr viral infection. Whatever the cause, it has occurred, and at times in epidemic proportions. It was first described in 1984 by two physicians in Incline Village, Nevada, when 300 of the residents of the small community developed "non-stop" flu.

Fatigue is a common symptom, but who isn't tired at times? As many as 25% of patients coming into a doctor's office will complain of fatigue. But how many have the chronic fatigue syndrome "disease?" Most of these patients are not "chronically" fatigued, and of those that are, only 1% to 3% may have CFS, according to the Centers for Disease Control. Even this small percentage produces many patients who are chronically fatigued and depressed. The question often asked is, "Are they sick because they are depressed, or are they depressed because they are sick?" More than likely, it is the latter.

Since the cause is not known and the disease is hard to diagnose, treatment is difficult and hard to evaluate. One physician is following 1,000 patients whom she believes to have CFS. She has reported that 50% have recovered after being treated with an anti-fungal drug and placed on a sugar-free diet.

If your teenage son reads this article, he will probably try to avoid mowing the lawn by claiming "chronic fatigue syndrome." If he tries it, cut out his sugar snacks and candy bars, and start the mower for him.

OTITIS MEDIA

The child screaming as the airplane ascends to 10,000 feet, the adult having a severe earache after SCUBA diving, the infant with a high fever, the boy with a hearing loss—all may be suffering from problems in the middle ear.

Our ears are divided into three parts: the external, the middle, and the inner ear. The "ear" that we can see on the side of our head and the ear canal together make up the external ear. The canal may become plugged with cerumen (wax) which must be washed out or removed. Occasionally the canal can develop an infection and antibiotics will be required.

The inner ear contains the cochlea (the hearing organ which converts the sound waves to nerve impulses), and the semicircular canals which give us our sense of balance. Fortunately, infections in this area are rare, but complications can be severe when they do occur.

It is the middle ear which gives children and adults the greatest problems. Otitis media or infection of the middle ear, is the second most common infection in childhood, after upper respiratory infections (colds). Seventy percent of children will suffer from otitis media during their first three years. If left untreated, the infection will usually clear in 10 to 14 days, but the resulting pain, fever and complications can be avoided. Before antibiotics were available, an infection of the middle ear would often follow a sore throat or common cold. First a child experiences fever, then an earache which increases daily, and finally relief when the eardrum ruptures and the fluid drains from the ear.

As these infections could occur several times a year during childhood, the complications (before antibiotics) were many and serious. Permanently ruptured eardrums, loss or scarring of the ossicles (the bones in the middle ear which transmit the sound), mastoiditis (an infection of the skull just behind the ear), and abscesses of the brain, were all possible long term complications of otitis media.

With the introduction of penicillin and the other antibiotics, the whole problem changed for the better. Today, at the first signs of fever or the child pulling at the ear or complaining of ear pain, parents usually see the pediatrician or family physician for diagnosis and treatment. If otitis media is diagnosed, antibiotics are usually prescribed. Today's drugs of choice are amoxicillin (a type of penicillin), Bactrim or Septra, and erythromycin. The choice is determined after considering any possible allergies and by the preference of the doctor. Other medications such as decongestants and antihistamines may be given to help the fluid drain down the eustachian tube. After 72 hours the child should be examined again to determine if the infection is clearing. If it is not, then a change in the antibiotics or a possible myringotomy (a small incision in the ear drum to drain the fluid) may be indicated.

With recurrent infections, fluid may continue to be present behind the ear drum and an operation to put a very small plastic tube through the drum can be performed by an ENT specialist. These tubes may remain in place for 6 to 12 months and are helpful in preventing future infections as well as restoring the child's hearing.

Why is otitis media so common in children and yet rare in adults? The answer lies in the size and the angle of the eustachian tube, the canal of internal skin that connects the middle ear to the back of the throat. This tube allows you to "pop" your ears when you drive up or down a mountain. The air pressure outside the body must equal the air pressure behind the ear drum if the drum is to retain its correct curves and work properly. If you have reach a high elevation and are unable to equalize the middle ear by having air come through the eustachian tube, the drum will swell outward and produce severe pain. The treatment is to yawn or swallow, which helps to open the tubes. If you have a cold and can not equalize your ears, return to a lower elevation immediately.

When a child develops a throat infection, the bacteria can travel up the small, short tube to the middle ear and spread the infection. Worse yet is when the eustachian tube becomes infected and is swollen shut. This prevents the infected fluid from draining into the throat, and causes the ear drum to bulge outward and finally rupture—ouch!

As a child grows older the eustachian tube grows larger and the chance of it closing from an infection is reduced; however, middle ear infections can still occur in adults, and treatment with the same antibiotics is the normal procedure.

NEVER, NEVER go SCUBA diving if you have a cold! Even an adult's eustachian tubes will swell and make it difficult to descend during a dive. Even if you are able to "pop" your ears and make it to the bottom, you may have a harder time getting back to the surface. As you ascend, the pressurized air behind the drum will expand. If it cannot escape through the eustachian tube, severe ear pain will result. The air will either rupture the eardrum or "blow open" the tube which will result in a nosebleed.

I repeat, *never* SCUBA dive with a cold!

Middle ear infections and problems occur more frequently in children than adults, but no one is immune. If you or your child develop a fever and/or an earache, see your family physician or pediatrician right away. Proper treatment can save you considerable pain and possible long-term complications such as permanent hearing loss.

COPD

Regardless of your age, when your doctor starts talking about COPD, pay attention. Your life may depend on it. Although it is the fifth leading cause of death in the U.S., COPD is preventable!

Chronic Obstructive Pulmonary Disease (COPD) is the term used to describe the condition of obstruction of the passage of air into and out of the lungs. When a person is unable to effectively get enough oxygen into the lungs, the body's systems begin to fail and the patient will ultimately die.

COPD is most often caused by either chronic bronchitis, emphysema or a combination of the two. Asthmatic bronchitis and bronchiectasis (a chronic lung infection) may at times contribute to the disease, but they are not as common. Chronic bronchitis is defined as a daily cough with production of sputum for three consecutive months. Remember that terrible cough from the flu which just wouldn't quit—one type of chronic bronchitis. Emphysema occurs when the tiny air sacs (alveoli) in the lung begin to break down and form larger sacs which are not as efficient in diffusing the oxygen from the air into the blood. The appearance of a patient with emphysema is a clue to the diagnosis. They are "barrel chested" because their lungs have expanded as much as possible in order to obtain more oxygen.

The causes of chronic bronchitis and emphysema are familiar to all of us: smoking and environmental factors. Cigarettes, the number one cause of illness in our country, is the major cause of chronic bronchitis and emphysema. "Smoker's cough," with the morning sputum, is a warning sign that a person is headed down the path to COPD, pulmonary disability, and an early death. Air pollutants, such as the SMOG in Los Angeles, can play a significant part in developing these lung conditions.

It takes many years to develop emphysema, and quitting smoking or avoiding air pollutants are the first and most important steps in preventing COPD. These steps may stop the progression of the disease and avoid the long term consequences of weakness and inability to breathe.

Once COPD has occurred, the treatments include eliminating the irritating agents (cigarettes and air pollutants), the use of drugs to open the air passages to the lungs, and finally the use of oxygen in an effort to increase the oxygen level in the blood.

Even when mild COPD has developed, quitting smoking can add five or more years to the patient's life by removing the irritation. Drugs become extremely important in increasing the air entering the lungs. Around each bronchus (air passage) in the lung is a small muscle which, if relaxed, will allow more air to pass into the lung. The drugs which can accomplish this are a group known as the beta-adrenergic agents, and include the brand names Proventil, Ventolin, Alupent, Bronkosol, and Brethaire. Usually they are administered by the use of an inhaler which gives a measured dose with each compression.

The drug theophylline not only relaxes the bronchiolar muscles, but it is also believed to improve the strength of the diaphragm and thereby improve the function of the lung. Corticosteroids are used when the patient no longer responds to the beta-adrenergic agents or to theophylline. The steroids reduce the edema and swelling around the air passages, but the side effects can be life threatening and the drugs must be used with caution.

Oxygen treatment becomes vital in the final stages of COPD. As the oxygen level in the blood continues to fall, despite the use of medications, the patient will become weaker and unable to do even simple tasks without being "short of breath." The administration of oxygen by a mask or by "plastic prongs" to the nose will increase the concentration of oxygen in the lung. This in turn will improve the oxygen level in the blood, and the patient will regain some of his strength. It is now recommended that the patient have continuous low-flow oxygen rather than have it only for 12 or 15 hours at a time. Survival appears to increase by months when the oxygen is constant.

Having chronic obstructive pulmonary disease (COPD) is not a pleasant way to end one's years. One sure way to avoid it is to stop smoking. Yes, COPD *is* preventable!

ADHESIONS

When small scars result from nature healing the nicks and scrapes of our skin, we rarely complain about the resulting scar tissue. However this same healing process inside the abdomen, following an operation, can result in adhesions (internal scars) which can have troublesome side effects.

Many people know about or have experienced "adhesions in the belly" but what are they? Why do they occur? What kinds of troubles do they cause?

Adhesions are essentially scar formations within the abdomen and are nature's way of controlling infections, foreign bodies or intestinal injuries. Mother Nature had been at this job for hundreds of thousands of years before physicians came on the scene, and it was only those cave men (and cave women) who were able to form adhesions who survived and passed this natural ability on to their children.

Adhesions develop following any operation in the abdomen. Surgeries, such as those on the appendix, stomach, intestine or uterus, will produce adhesions as the body heals inside. Surgeons try to be very gentle with the inside organs as well as washing the blood, bile and other materials from the cavity, yet adhesions still form.

Other than surgery there are assorted causes of adhesion formation. Some adhesions, such as those formed by perforated ulcers, appendicitis and infections in women's fallopian tubes, can be reduced through early recognition and treatment.

If adhesions are a natural healing process, why worry about them? Abdominal adhesions are like ukulele strings stretching between the intestines or from the front of the abdomen to the back. The intestine can wrap itself around the adhesion blocking that portion of the bowel and preventing the food from passing through. This condition is called "intestinal obstruction." The obstructed portion of bowel will become larger and larger until a perforation or rupture of the bowel occurs with resultant infection, shock and death.

What are the symptoms of intestinal obstruction? The patient will experience nausea, then abdominal pain, and finally vomiting. The vomiting may occur in waves, being quiet for a while and then recurring like a storm. Everyone has experienced intestinal flu with these identical symptoms, but that does not indicate intestinal obstruction. However, if you have had abdominal surgery and the intense cramping and vomiting persists for more than an hour, then it is possible that an intestinal obstruction has developed. You should see your physician immediately.

Nature has been marvelous in protecting the human body with its healing processes but, perhaps the next time the body is designed, a little more time could be spent on preventing intestinal adhesions.

KIDDIE HERNIAS

Hernias in infants and children are a more serious problem than those in adolescents and adults. The physician's main worry regarding inguinal (groin) hernias is that bowel may become "stuck" (incarcerated) and that the blood supply to the bowel may then be cut off (strangulated), with resulting death of the bowel and death of the patient.

In young and older adults the hernias tend to enlarge slowly, causing pain and an inconvenience to the patient; however, only occasionally will they become incarcerated (stuck). This is not the case with infants and children. Several times a year, I'm called to the emergency room to evaluate a child with an incarcerated hernia (along with a frantic mother).

With infants and children, the cause of the hernia is a congenital (born with it) sac which extends from the abdominal cavity down the groin and into the scrotum. As the intestine slides down this sac, the infant experiences pain, cries, and alerts the mother to the hernia. A bulge is present in the groin and may extend into the scrotum. If gentle pressure on the bulge causes it to go "squish" back into the abdomen, then it is an uncomplicated hernia; on the other hand, if the swelling refuses to "squish," the hernia is incarcerated (or stuck) and an emergency exists.

The surgery to correct an infant's hernia is not as difficult as it is with an adult. After the baby is anesthetized (put to sleep), an inch incision is made in the skin crease above the pubic bone. Then, after going through a half inch of fat, a small nick is made in the fascia (stringy fibers) that lays over the hernia sac. The sac is separated from the spermatic cord (the vessels going to the testicle), opened, and the intestine is pushed back into the abdomen. Next, it is tied with suture (thread). The fascia and skin are sutured closed and, PRESTO, the operation is over!

In contrast, when the hernia has been stuck for several hours, there are more complications. The intestine will be edematous (swollen) and may even be necrotic (dead). Anesthesia is harder and more dangerous. Usually the incision is larger. But I find the hardest part is the dissection of the sac, which is edematous and has the consistency of wet Kleenex. If the bowel has a "dead" area, another incision on the abdomen must be made in order to remove the dead portion and connect the ends of the healthy intestine.

What I enjoy most about operating on children is that the next day they are running around as though nothing had happened! Adults will moan and groan for several days.

Most surgeons recommend that hernias in infants and children be repaired as soon as possible. Doing so may save an emergency operation that will create more stress for the child, the mother and the surgeon.

LUMPS

My friend, Kathi, came into my office and was very concerned about a newly discovered lump in her scalp. It took her only a few seconds to find it for me on the back of her skull at the junction with her neck. She was relieved when I told her that most people have it, and that she wasn't going to die from it. It was the normal external occipital protuberance of the skull where five bony ridges on the skull converge.

I didn't tease Kathi about her worries because I can still remember in medical school my worries about several lumps which had me convinced I had only a few months to live. My first experience occurred during the second year of medical school in my pathology class. We were studying about cancers and their spread to lymph nodes. I nonchalantly felt my neck, AND FOUND SEVERAL LUMPS! The more I examined, the more nodes I found. I was in a cold sweat by the end of the class, and I stumbled to the outpatient department to be examined by a real doctor.

The resident asked me questions about past infections, weight loss, loss of sleep (all medical students lose weight and have no time to sleep). I knew that I was going to be diagnosed as having leukemia or something worse. Finally, he laughed at me and assured me that my lymph nodes were normal, resulting from many throat infections I had had as a child. Sheepishly, I went back to my next class.

Almost everyone will have several small, soft lymph nodes in the neck. Lymph nodes can also be felt in the armpits and in the groin. These are the body's first line of defense if an infection occurs. When the nodes become tender, hard or increase in size, it is time to see your doctor. These are warning signs that an infection or tumor is present.

My second experience began during the next year when I was in my orthopedic rotation, studying bones and their tumors. I should never have examined my right wrist. I found MORE LUMPS! I thought I had osteogenic sarcoma (a bone cancer) and would not be alive long enough to graduate from medical school. This time I went to the professor for my terminal diagnosis, and again was laughed at. I was informed that I had two ganglia of my wrist and they probably wouldn't bother me, let alone kill me.

A ganglion is a cyst that arises off the capsule surrounding a joint or a tendon. It is common around the wrists and ankles. If the ganglion becomes too large, it may become painful or interfere with motion of the joint or tendon. The treatment is usually aspiration with a needle and syringe, and if it recurs, then surgical excision is necessary.

Another lump which most of us have, some more than others, is the xyphoid bone at the bottom of our chest bone. The chest bone in front is actually three bones: the manubrium at the top, the sternum in the middle, and the xyphoid at the bottom.

The xyphoid is pointed and is located in the area referred to as "the pit of the stomach." Sometimes the pointed end sticks forward (especially in women following pregnancies) and can be of great concern to the patient. Reassurance and explanation are all that is necessary.

Lumps on our bodies should be of concern to us, and we should understand their causes. Knowing about these four examples will relieve some of your worries. I still have my ganglia, partially because they have not bothered me, but also to remind me to be more understanding when someone comes to my office worried about a lump which turns out to be normal.

THYROID

The thyroid gland is located in the mid-portion of the neck just below and to either side of your "Adam's apple." Actually, the "Adam's apple" is the thyroid cartilage which surrounds the voice box. This gland is very important for our general well-being, but for many individuals it can be a problem.

The function of the thyroid is to produce a hormone which is the "additive" in the gasoline of your body. When there is an over-production of the hormone it is called a "hyperthyroid state." The result is that the metabolism of the body accelerates with a resulting increase in the body's temperature, fatigue of the muscles, excitability of the nerves, and loss of weight.

The "hypothyroid" state occurs when the thyroid gland does not produce enough thyroid hormone to keep the body's engines running properly, and an overweight condition can result (this is only one of the many reasons for being overweight).

The thyroid gland can become swollen because of a lack of iodine in the diet. This condition, goiter, is common throughout the mid-western states due to an iodine deficient diet. However, the ocean is abundant with iodine and a true goiter is very rare among those who live near oceans.

Occasionally a single lump or nodule will occur in the gland and there is concern that cancer is present. Fortunately, most thyroid lumps are not cancerous and certain tests are used to exclude this possibility. The first test is a radio-isotope "scan" of the thyroid gland to determine if the nodule is working and is "hot." Hot nodules are rarely cancerous, but a "cold" nodule warrants greater concern. If it is "cold" the next procedure is an ultrasound exam of the thyroid gland to determine whether or not this "cold" nodule is cystic (filled with fluid) or whether it is solid which would increase the chances of diagnosing it as cancer.

A needle biopsy of the nodule will answer the question, "Is it a cyst, or is it a tumor?" If cystic, fluid will be drawn off and the lump will disappear. If solid, the needle will remove a small piece of the tissue that can then be examined by the pathologist to determine if a cancer is present.

If a benign (not a cancerous) nodule is found, the patient will be started on high doses of thyroid medication to "suppress" the thyroid gland and to see if the nodule disappears. If the nodule does not change, then an operation to remove the nodule and part of the thyroid gland is indicated.

Although cancer of the thyroid gland is uncommon, there are three or four cases treated annually at Maui Memorial Hospital. Fortunately, thyroid cancer, when diagnosed early, is curable in 90% to 95% of patients.

Last of all, there is a concern about thyroid conditions resulting from x-ray treatment. During the past 10 years there has been considerable investigation of individuals exposed to x-ray treatment as children. Thirty or 40 years ago it was common to treat enlarged tonsils, acne, or head and neck problems with high doses of x-ray. Fortunately, this procedure is no longer practiced. Unfortunately, many of these individuals, who are now young and middle-aged adults, are developing both benign and malignant tumors of the thyroid gland.

I would certainly advise any reader, who as a child received prolonged x-ray treatment for these conditions, to contact a physician for a thyroid examination. Early detection of this cancer is an important factor in its excellent cure rate.

ENLARGEMENT OF THE MALE BREAST—GYNECOMASTIA

About once a week a very worried mother will bring her embarrassed teenage son into my office for an examination. The problem is that the boy has noticed a painful lump in one of his breasts and the mother is worried about the possibility of breast cancer. The examination will usually reveal a tender lump about the size of a nickel behind the nipple and, if the rest of the exam is normal, I can reassure the mother and son that this is a benign (not cancerous) condition called gynecomastia (meaning woman's breast) and that it will usually disappear when he finishes puberty.

Gynecomastia develops in about 60-70% of normal boys during puberty, the ages of 12 to 15, and usually does not cause symptoms. However it may occur during later years and be a significant problem to diagnose and treat.

The cause of gynecomastia is believed to be an excess of estrogens (the female hormone) over the androgens (the male hormone) in the boy or man. Yes, in the normal man there are female hormones at work, but don't tell any "Primo Warriors." During puberty there is an increase in both the male and female hormones, and the elevated estrogen may stimulate a small amount of breast development, or gynecomastia. This clears when the male hormones (androgens) increase.

In older men, the physician must evaluate the patient for other conditions causing the breast enlargement. Breast cancer must be checked for first. Although rare in men, it accounts for 0.2% of male cancers and is very deadly. Tumors of the adrenal glands and testes can produce estrogens causing breast enlargement. Hyperthyroidism (an overactive thyroid gland) and cirrhosis of the liver may also cause gynecomastia. However the most common cause of breast enlargement in the adult male is a "side effect" of a drug that he is taking. Several commonly used drugs may have this side effect: Valium, Tagamet, reserpine, digitalis, methyldopa and estrogens, to name some.

Treatment of gynecomastia depends upon the cause and the degree of the breast enlargement. In the adult, the medications causing the problem should be changed, if possible. In other cases, the condition can be corrected, such as when a tumor develops or with hyperthyroidism.

In the young male, the swelling usually subsides with time, but ice-packs and aspirin will relieve the tenderness. Occasionally the breast enlargement may be so great that it is embarrassing to the boy and he will refuse to participate in sports. In such cases, surgery is indicated in order to reduce the size of the breast so that it is normal in appearance.

Mother, if your teenage son has a small tender lump behind the nipple, it is probably a normal part of puberty; however, if a lump appears in an adult male, it is a more serious matter and a thorough investigation should be performed by his physician.

A GIRL'S BREAST LUMP

Gail (not her real name), age 14, was brought into my office by her worried mother. During a physical exam the previous week, a doctor discovered that she had a large breast tumor. After a mammogram had confirmed her tumor, she now needed a breast biopsy and a possible mastectomy (removal of the breast).

Cancers in the adolescent breast are exceedingly rare, but benign tumors are not. A discussion of these two types of tumors will help mothers and their teenage daughters.

Puberty in girls usually begins around 10-12 years of age. The pituitary gland at the base of the brain secretes the hormone FSH (follicle-stimulating hormone) which causes the immature ovaries to develop, and they in turn produce estrogens. The estrogens induce the growth and maturation of the breasts.

At about age 10 to 12, glandular tissue will begin to develop beneath the nipples. Between 11 to 13 years of age, the breast will show enlargement with further increase in the glandular tissue. By 14 to 17 the breasts will have reached their full adolescent size. Frequently the breasts will not develop at the same rate and one side may be much larger, appearing to harbor a tumor while in actuality it is normal.

Probably the greatest danger to the developing breast is an over anxious surgeon. A biopsy of the mammary bud beneath the nipple will stunt the growth of that breast. Experience and good judgment become very important in making the decision to biopsy a young girl's breast.

While a cyst is uncommon in the adolescent breast, a fibroadenoma (benign type of tumor) is not. Several times a year I am asked to examine a young girl who will later be found to have a fibroadenoma. These tumors are most common during the second and third decades of life, but can occur any time after puberty. The lumps are usually firm and smooth, ranging in size from a pea to a large orange. Mammograms are usually not indicated, but an ultrasound examination of the breast can provide valuable information without the risk of radiation. An operation to excise only the fibroadenoma will cure the patient and will leave the breast normal in appearance.

A rare and most unusual tumor that can occur in the adolescent breast is a cystosarcoma phyllodes. It grows quite rapidly and at times is mistaken for a giant fibroadenoma. However, the cystosarcoma phyllodes can recur locally if not completely excised, and 5% may metastasize (spread to other parts of the body) and kill the patient. Neither of these complications occurs with the fibroadenoma.

Children, adolescents and adults may develop another rare cancer termed a juvenile or secretory carcinoma. Patients have ranged in age from 3 to 73. The recovery rate is very favorable, and most patients are cured with either a wide excision or a mastectomy.

A lump in a young girl's breast will cause a great deal of worry to both the mother and the daughter. An early trip, rather than a prolonged delay, to the family physician or pediatrician will relieve their minds and possibly avoid horrible consequences.

Gail's biopsy was benign and the giant fibroadenoma was removed, leaving a normal appearing breast. Gail, her family and her surgeon were all overjoyed with the final diagnosis and outcome.

SHIGELLA

The other day, a patient suffering from vomiting and diarrhea brought back memories of Maui's greatest epidemic, some 20 years ago. I had been practicing surgery on Maui for two years and, like all the Maui doctors, I helped treat the emergency room patients.

Friday night, August 17, 1970, we began to have an unusual number of patients coming to the ER complaining of diarrhea. By Saturday morning the doctors' offices were crowded with very uncomfortable patients, all with the same symptoms of vomiting and diarrhea.

The State Health Department was contacted and they, in turn, called for help from the Communicable Disease Center (CDC) in Atlanta, Georgia. A team of epidemiologists was on the next plane headed to Maui. By the time the team arrived the epidemic was abating and Shigella Sonnei had been cultured as the offending bacteria. It was exciting to watch the CDC team do their detective work and discover how the epidemic had spread.

Shigellosis is now a rather rare disease on Maui but in 1970 there had been a rising number of cases with 55 being reported in July of that year. An outbreak of shigellosis had been seen in the area of Kapuna, just past Waihee, during the first week of August.

The epidemic, however, was island-wide so the CDC started looking at all possible causes. The water supply was eliminated because of the unlikely chance that the numerous different water supplies from Lahaina to Hana had been contaminated at the same time.

The likely source was food, but which one? The two dairy farms were investigated and the milk was found to be safe.

Then it was discovered that a large number of patients were Hawaiians or part-Hawaiian and most had been to a luau before becoming ill. Detailed investigation in the Hana area revealed that almost all the patients had eaten poi which had been delivered on Friday. Taking this information and applying it island-wide revealed that, indeed, the contaminated food was probably poi. Poi is a carbohydrate staple of the Hawaiian diet which is made from the taro plant. Tourists complain that it tastes like wallpaper paste.

The bacteria could no longer be cultured from the poi since it becomes acidic as it ferments, and the acid kills the bacteria. The epidemiologists checked and cultured the employees of the only poi factory on the island but none had Shigellosis. It was decided that contaminated taro grown in Kapuna, which was having a local outbreak of Shigellosis, infected the entire supply delivered to all of Maui that fateful Friday.

A review by the CDC team of doctors and ER records showed that there were more than 600 cases of Shigellosis that weekend making it the largest epidemic of Shigellosis ever reported in the United States! The complete report of the CDC team was published in the *American Journal of Epidemiology* (Vol 96, No. 1, 1972).

For me, Maui is still the most wonderful place in the world to live, and I still enjoy eating poi (once in a while) at a luau. The epidemic, however, pointed out that the safety of the food we eat requires a tremendous amount of continuing effort by the Department of Health. I tip my hat to them.

CAUSES OF STROKES

When people hear that someone has had a "stroke" they think of paralysis and heart problems. They are only half right. A stroke can cause paralysis (and many other ills) but it results from a condition in the brain, not in the heart.

There are 500,000 new cases of strokes a year in the U.S., and of those, 160,000 die. The remainder of the patients have varying degrees of paralysis, partial blindness, memory or thought loss, and sometimes no problems at all.

So what is a stroke? It is the result of injuries to the brain. The brain is similar to a complex computer with millions of wires, brain cells called neurons. While a computer needs electricity, the brain cells require oxygen which is carried by blood. If you turn off the electricity to a computer, it ceases to work. If the blood is blocked from a part of the brain, that part will stop working and will usually die, although the patient continues to live.

As each part of the brain has a definite function—memory, thought process, vision, hearing, motor function, sensation—a loss of that area will cause a corresponding deficit. Because the motor function areas of the brain (those moving the muscles of our body) are so large, most strokes will result in some degree of muscle paralysis.

There are two reasons why blood and oxygen fail to reach the brain. The first is clogging of the arteries, either by thrombosis (a blood clot or arteriosclerosis blocking the artery) or an embolis (a blood clot forming elsewhere in the body and floating to the brain). The second reason is a cerebral hemorrhage, or bleeding in the brain. When an artery bursts in or around the brain, the blood clot compresses the adjacent brain so that the blood can no longer reach the brain cells; hence the cells die. Approximately 80% of strokes are caused by a clogging of the arteries and 20% by bleeding.

There are three medical problems which increase the risk of a stroke, and if avoided will decrease that risk. Hypertension (high blood pressure) has long been known to be a significant contributor to a stroke. The energetic campaign to have people know their blood pressure, and to control it when it is high, has resulted in a decrease in the incidence of strokes during the last 20 years. A high cholesterol (over 200) is a risk for arteriosclerosis with resulting strokes and heart attacks. Finally, diabetes causes both arteriosclerosis and weakening in the arteries with resulting bleeding.

Do you know your blood pressure, cholesterol and blood sugar levels? If not, you may be risking a stroke which could be avoided with proper medical care.

WARNING SIGNS OF STROKES

How do you know if a stroke is threatening either you or a loved one? Are there warning signs which could alert you to seek medical care in order to prevent a stroke from occurring?

Approximately 35% of strokes are caused by thrombosis or clotting of the large arteries in the neck. Most people at immediate risk will have warning signs before the stroke occurs. As the artery is closing off, and less blood is getting to the brain, the individual may experience numbness, tingling, weakness in the face or in an extremity. The complaint will last only a few minutes and is called a TIA (transient ischemic attack). As only one or two of these TIA's may occur before a major stroke, it is important to seek evaluation immediately so that the proper studies can be performed.

Another warning sign that the arteries in the neck are closing up is the sound of a bruit (abnormal sound or murmur). Your doctor can hear this with his stethoscope as he listens over the artery. The sound is similar to the hiss when you kink a garden hose.

Once a thrombosis of the carotid artery (the large artery in the neck) is suspected, there are several investigative procedures available to make the diagnosis and to determine if surgery or medication is necessary. The most commonly used test is a Doppler ultrasound of the neck. Pictures are taken of the arteries by using ultrasound waves. This is a good, safe screening test which can determine if a major blockage is present. If surgery is being considered, then a carotid angiogram will be necessary. This is an x-ray study where dye is injected into the carotid arteries so that they can be studied closely. There is a small risk of causing a stroke with the procedure, so it is not performed unless absolutely necessary.

If the studies show that the artery is blocked 80% or more, or if the patient has had a TIA, then a carotid endarterectomy (surgery on the carotid artery) is recommended. The surgeon becomes a very delicate plumber by opening the pipe to the brain (the carotid artery) and carefully removing the plaque of cholesterol which is plugging it. Rare complications can occur with the operation, but the mortality rate is less than 2%. Following surgery, the TIA's should disappear and the patient's chances of developing a stroke are greatly reduced. This operation cannot be performed after a stroke has occurred, as it may intensify the symptoms.

Following thrombosis, embolism is the next most common cause of a stroke. Embolism occurs when a blood clot, that forms elsewhere in the body, breaks loose and is carried by the blood to the brain where it blocks an artery. The most common area for the embolis to form is in the heart when atrial fibrillation is present. Atrial fibrillation is an abnormal beating of one of the chambers of the heart. The physician will usually prescribe an anticoagulant medicine to prevent such a clot from occurring.

Only about 5% of strokes are caused by the bleeding from a ruptured berry aneurysm, but, unfortunately, these strokes usually occur in younger people. Aneurysms are weakened areas of an artery, and in the brain they look like berries hanging from a branch. When the aneurysm ruptures there is usually a large hemorrhage with compression of the brain, coma and death. Occasionally the berry aneurysm will leak for days or even weeks before the rupture occurs. This leakage will cause a headache which should alert the patient and his doctor that something is wrong. Headaches which occur with exertion, or for the first time after age 35, or "the worst headache ever" are all warning signs of a possible leaking aneurysm. Quick referral to a neurosurgeon is the only chance to avert a major stroke.

Although some strokes cannot be prevented, it is known that controlling your blood pressure, cholesterol and diabetes will lessen your risk. If you have numbness or weakness lasting only a few minutes or an unusually severe headache, see your physician immediately.

5 Injuries

DANGERS OF BARBECUING

Barbecue alert! I thought I was familiar with all the dangers involved in the great American pasttime of outside barbecuing, but I discovered a brand new one last week. We have all heard of some dangers: never barbecue inside the house because of the dangers of the carbon monoxide which is produced; watch out for small children around the fire as they like to touch the metal or the hot grill; NEVER, NEVER use gasoline to start the coals as the explosion may send you and your guests to the hospital. But what about the wire brush that is used to clean last week's grease off the grill? Do we need to beware of this "invaluable" tool?

I was called to the emergency room to see Ken because the ER doctor was worried that he might have appendicitis. For the previous four days Ken had been having abdominal pain, unlike anything he had experienced before. The pain had begun in the "pit" of his stomach and then had moved to the lower part of the abdomen, which was typical for appendicitis. But the pain had not increased during the next several days, which is not typical. There had been neither vomiting nor fever, and the white blood count was normal, again not typical for appendicitis. Another important consideration about Ken was that he had had surgery on his stomach 10 years ago, but he did not know if the appendix had been removed at that time.

The pain in his abdomen had not improved by the next

morning, so I ordered a barium enema x-ray of the colon (the large intestine). If the appendix (which is attached to the colon) filled with the barium, then appendicitis was unlikely. The appendix didn't fill, so appendicitis was a strong possibility! Ken was told of the possible diagnosis and the risks of the surgery. He agreed to an operation.

I still had my doubts about the diagnosis, so I made Ken's incision different and larger than the usual one for an appendectomy. I began looking for the appendix, and guess what? The appendix was gone. It had been removed at the time of his stomach surgery 10 years ago. Something else had to be causing his pain, so I began an "exploration" of his intestines.

The first thing I looked for was a Meckle's diverticulum. This is a congenital (present at birth) pouch on the small intestine, and at times it can become infected, just like appendicitis. I began running the bowel through my gloved hands when I discovered a *thin black wire sticking through the wall of the intestine*! Now I have been a surgeon for 30 years, but I had never seen this before! I removed the wire and saved it for the pathologist. Then I examined the remainder of the bowel and found *another thin black wire*, again sticking through the bowel's wall. I sent it to the lab, also. No other problems were found in Ken's abdomen so I sutured the incision and the operation was over.

The "$64,000 Question" was "Where did the wires come from?" Ken's friends starting discussing the possibilities and remembered that someone at their condominium had found a wire in a hamburger cooked on the outside barbecue. Ken remembered having a couple hamburgers from that grill the night before his pains had started. The hunt was on for the barbecue brush!

The next day, Ken showed me the suspect brush which had been brought in by his friends. Two-thirds of the wires had broken off and those that remained appeared to match the two which I had taken from Ken's intestine!

For those of you who enjoy barbecuing, I offer the following advice: do not use barbecue coals in the house, never use gasoline to start the fire, keep children away from the grill, and throw away any wire brushes showing rust or wear. Better yet, clean the cold grill with a rough plastic scouring pad!

SPLENIC INJURIES

Sally is a strong young lady, but it is still hard for me to believe that she had walked the mile from her apartment to the doctor's office with the pain she was experiencing. The night before, she had been struck in her abdomen during a fight, and severe pain developed. Rather than call an ambulance and "inconvenience anyone," she waited until morning and walked to the office despite the pains in her abdomen and left shoulder. Her doctor sent her to my office and, after examining her, I immediately called 911 for the ambulance and admitted her to the hospital with a diagnosis of a ruptured spleen!

The spleen is an organ in the body about which much is known but still more is being learned every year. During fetal development (that time before we are born) the spleen produces red and white blood cells. Following birth, it serves two important functions: being a source of antibody formation (which helps fight infections) and, equally important, acting as a filter to cleanse the blood. Its normal size is about that of a person's clenched fist. It is located in the abdomen beneath the left diaphragm and is protected by the lower ribs. During surgery, doctors comment that the spleen usually looks red and bloody, but the pathologists talk about its red and white pulp. The red pulp is actually the many blood vessels which act as the filter. The white pulp is the collection of the white blood cells, lymphocytes, plasma cells and macrophages, which produce the antibodies and help clean the blood.

Is the spleen a vital organ, essential to our survival, or is it one that can be casually removed and discarded, like the appendix? Because of injury or illness, many people have had their spleens removed and have lived normal lives. On the other hand, certain individuals, especially children, need their spleens in order to fight deadly infections.

Splenectomies (surgical removal of the spleen) have been performed in the U. S. for over 150 years. The first operations were done to remove those injured in fights and accidents. Later it was learned that enlarged, diseased spleens could be removed with the patient receiving some temporary relief.

One of the functions of the spleen is to "clean" the blood by trapping and destroying old blood cells and platelets (small particles in our blood which help it to clot). In one disease, ITP (immune thrombocytopenic purpura), the spleen runs amuck and destroys too many platelets, with bruising and bleeding of the patient occurring. If the patient is not helped with steroid medications, then removing the spleen will usually cure this disease.

Forty years ago the spleen was considered to be more of a liability than an important organ of the body. If it was injured even slightly during an operation, it was quickly removed rather than repaired. Then in 1952 it was discovered that there were many children dying of pneumonia after having had their spleens removed. Investigations showed that patients after a splenectomy, and especially children, had a reduction in their immune system and therefore were more susceptible to infections.

With this new information, surgeons make every effort to repair and save spleens which might have been injured in an accident. This is not an easy task. The spleen has the consistency of uncooked liver, and sutures tend to tear through the tissue and cause even more bleeding. With their best efforts, surgeons are able to save only 50% of injured spleens. When the spleen must be removed, the patient is given antibiotics and a pneumonia vaccination in order to reduce the risks of serious infections.

Sally was given fluids and blood to raise her blood pressure and bring her blood count back to normal. A CAT scan (a special x-ray exam) of her spleen revealed that it had been badly torn and that there was a large blood clot surrounding it. Because the bleeding had not stopped, Sally was taken to the operating room and a surgical exploration performed. Indeed, the spleen was still bleeding and the injury so great that a repair was not possible. The artery and veins supplying the spleen were tied with silk, cut, and the pieces of spleen removed. After surgery, Sally received antibiotics and a pneumonia vaccination. Her recovery was rapid and she was discharged at the end of the week.

The spleen has proved to be an important organ, especially vital to children. Its functions continue to be discovered and, as immunology becomes more significant in future medicine, the spleen will probably be shown to serve a very important role.

HYPOTHERMIA

Today, after spending a wonderfully warm day at the beach, I found it hard to believe that a week ago my family and I were in Telluride, Colorado where two feet of snow was still on the ground and our major concern was to survive the elements. We have become "soft" after living on Maui for so long, particularly since we do not have to constantly fight the weather (except for an occasional Kona storm). On the other hand, half of the people on the Mainland must adjust their entire living customs (clothes, homes and autos) in order to live through the winter months.

The harshness of the elements was made vivid to me in Telluride when I helped care for a young skier who was injured in an avalanche. He was a "hot shot" skier who was skiing in an "out of bounds" area when suddenly the snow beneath him gave way. The avalanche carried him about 1/4 mile before he (and the avalanche) fell 100 feet over a cliff. Fortunately two of his fellow skiers had not been caught in the avalanche, were able to keep up with him, and spotted where he finally stopped. One skier went to get help from the ski patrol while the other went to dig out his injured friend.

I was at the Telluride Clinic when the call came in that we were to receive an avalanche victim. In anticipation of having to treat hypothermia, the nurse immediately placed several blankets into the autoclave in order to heat them quickly. The victim arrived by helicopter, already in traction for a fractured leg. His first temperature at the clinic was 94 degrees which signals the start of hypothermia. We cut off his cold wet clothes and wrapped him in the warm blankets. His temperature returned to normal within 30 minutes. By that time his other fractures had been stabilized and he was ready to be transferred to the nearest hospital in Montrose, Colorado.

What is hypothermia and when does it become dangerous? Hypothermia literally means "low temperature" and is the condition when the body's temperature falls below 95 degrees Fahrenheit. Mild hypothermia ranges from 95 to 90 degrees, moderate hypothermia from 89-79 degrees, deep hypothermia 77-68 degrees, and profound hypothermia occurs below 67 degrees. The major complaint of mild hypothermia is that of shivering as the body attempts to produce heat with rapid muscular contractions. With moderate hypothermia (89-79 degrees) the brain becomes clouded and a coma can occur. The heart also slows its rate and becomes very irritable. As the temperature drops, the heart may develop fibrillation and stop.

Fortunately hypothermia is unknown on Maui. It will take another 11 months of warm Maui beaches before I'll be ready to return to the ski slopes of Colorado.

SPINAL CORD INJURY

Accidents occur constantly and they always pose a danger to our lives or the lives of those we love. I have written before about the injuries from burns and automobile accidents where a momentary lapse of judgment can result in a lifetime of pain, disfigurement or even death. Now I want to focus on spinal cord injuries. Across our country 50% of spinal cord injuries are due to automobile accidents.

On Maui there appears to be a higher incidence of these injuries due to the "paradise playground" in which we live, rather than to the automobile. I would estimate that the majority of patients with spinal cord problems seen at Maui Memorial Hospital sustain their injury from swimming, either when the patient has been rolled on the beach by a large wave or when someone has carelessly dived into a swimming pool or a mountain stream.

Other types of injuries that can damage the spinal cord include severe falls, gunshot injuries to the spine (fortunately rare on Maui), and infections of the spinal cord (such as meningitis). One patient injured himself when he fell from a bar stool and broke his neck.

Our spinal cord is only a bundle of very soft wires (called neurons) that carry the impulses from the body to the brain and then back to the other parts of the body. It is an extremely complex and delicate bundle of fibers that can be injured easily.

Evolution has placed this bundle of nerve fibers in a flexible bony structure, called the spine. For most animals this "spine" adequately protects the delicate network. Evolution has not, however, developed our spines to withstand the forces of an automobile accident or of diving into the shallow end of a swimming pool, so spinal injuries occur.

What usually happens is that the vertebrae (those individual bones in the spine) are dislocated on each other and a shearing or squeezing of the spinal cord results. If the injury is severe enough, the spinal cord may be severed; however, a lesser injury may produce only a serious bruising that can either clear or, with swelling from the injury, progress on to the death of the spinal cord at that point. Death of the spinal cord at any level prevents the brain's nerve impulses from passing beyond that point. Hence the patient will be paralyzed below the point of the injury.

Depending upon where the injury has occurred, physicians classify the patient as either quadriplegic (four extremities paralyzed) or paraplegic (partially paralyzed). Injuries to the neck usually result in quadriplegia, that is, paralysis of both arms and both legs, while injuries to the lower spine result in the paralysis of only the legs.

The changes to the person suffering a spinal injury can be devastating. If he survives the injury (there may be many additional injuries to other organs at the same time), his life will never be the same. If the neck has been injured and he is quadriplegic (all four limbs paralyzed), then he will never be able to maintain himself; instead, he will always have to rely upon family, friends or special institutions for maintenance of his body. If he has paralysis of only the legs, then he may continue to have an active, productive life, but again must often rely upon help from others.

Besides the inability to care for oneself there are numerous additional medical problems such as hypotension (low blood pressure), constant bladder and kidney infections, and the most serious problem of recurrent skin ulcers. These ulcers form from pressure sores over bony prominences such as the hip bones.

When you and I sit on chairs, if we sit on a "bony area", the pain produced in the overlying skin causes us to readjust our position. This allows the blood to recirculate through the painful area and no damage occurs. But with a quadriplegic or paraplegic patient, there is no sensation in the skin. The patient does not feel the pain and, as a result, the pressure continues in this area shuts off the blood supply, and necrosis or tissue death occurs. The skin, underlying fat, and muscle sloughs away and the patient develops a skin ulcer.

It is a constant battle to prevent skin ulcers and serious kidney and bladder infections in order to help the patient maintain a good quality of life. It is a high price to pay for a moment of careless driving, the thrill of body surfing or a careless home accident. Only good judgment and common sense will help you avoid a needless spinal injury. Be careful!

HOUSEHOLD DANGERS

Gunshot wounds, third-degree burns, amputated fingers—all occur daily in the most dangerous place on earth. Lebanon? New York City? No, right in your own home. That's right, more injuries occur at home than in any other battlefield around the world. One of my readers asked me to write about lawn mower accidents, but there are many dangers around the "home-front battlefield" that demand attention.

Lawn mower accidents are always devastating and always preventable. There are three types of injuries: to the fingers, the toes, and from flying objects. The skin on the back of my neck crawls every time I hear of someone reaching under a lawn mower to dislodge the clumps of grass. Good-by fingers! Always turn off the engine before cleaning the blade! When someone mows the grass on a hillside while wearing sandals, good-by toes! Always wear protective shoes. Rocks and pieces of metal thrown by the blade of a mower are as dangerous as bullets and can cause serious injuries to anyone standing in the line of fire. Keep your lawn raked and free of those missiles.

The kitchen is probably the most dangerous room in the house. But that's no reason for the husband not to do the dishes. Burns from splattered grease, cuts from paring knives, lacerations from a dropped glass, hands ground in the garbage disposal, burns from touching hot pots and pans, fingers in the electric mixers, oven fires and hitting your head on the open cabinet door! No wonder my wife, Carole, wants to eat out so often.

The accidental poisoning of children is all too common. If you have small children, lock up all medicines and remove all those poisonous cleaning solutions from under the kitchen sink. Put them up high and away from little hands and mouths.

The workshop in the garage is a good source of injury and resulting income for the emergency room doctors. Don't use that Skill saw if you've been drinking; a split second mistake will cost you a finger or more. Wear glasses when you are drilling or sawing and you could save your eyes. A smashed finger from a hammer will hurt for several days, but fortunately the injury is usually mild.

Gunshot injuries are always tragic and frequently fatal. Far more people are killed at home by gunshot accidents than are killed by burglars. If you must have a gun at home, then be sure that it is not loaded and keep the ammunition safely locked up. Don't leave the key where the kids can find it or you will be asking for a tragedy.

Stepping on a needle in the rug is not fun, nor is a fall from a broken ladder. Using gasoline to start the barbecue and smoking in bed are sure ways to spend some time in a hospital bed recovering from second and third degree burns. Moving furniture without adequate help can put your back out of commission for several weeks.

All of these accidents and injuries can be prevented. Some require locking up the medicines and ammunition NOW. Others can be prevented by "thinking before you act." Remember, "Be it ever so dangerous, there's no place like home."

6 General Information

BILL AND HOSPICE

Bill, we will miss you. Your family and friends are relieved that you are finally free of your pain and free of the cancer which you had been fighting so bravely for such a long time. I hope that we were able to give you comfort and dispel the fears and loneliness of your last days and weeks. Bill, you might not have realized that you gave us a wonderful gift in return. You gave us the gift of allowing us to show our love and friendship. You gave purpose to our lives.

Your decision to spend your last days and weeks at home was the right one. With the help of Hospice Maui and the nurses from Home Health, it was possible for family and friends to give you compassionate care in the familiar surroundings of your home. We all must face those final days and, if we are not fortunate to go quickly, then most of us would prefer to spend those weeks and days at home rather than in even the best of hospitals. Because of this need, Hospice Maui was formed.

The Hospice movement was reborn in London in the late 1960's and led by Dr. Cicely Saunders. She recognized a need to treat terminal patients in a more compassionate way and, at the same time, keep them free of pain. During the Middle Ages, hospices were maintained by religious orders and were often for the care of terminal patients. During the last 100 years, as physicians became more successful in curing patients and discharging them from the hospital, the need for facilities to care for terminal patients diminished; however, the dying patients who remained in the hospital were often treated with fluids into their veins, tubes in their noses and painful injections to relieve the pain of their cancer. Worse yet was the loneliness of a hospital room and the absence of friends and family. Dr. Saunders set out to correct these problems when she opened St. Christopher's Hospice in southeast London.

The major principles of the hospice approach are to "treat the patient and not the disease," and "to maximize the quality of life when the quantity of life cannot be extended." The first goal is to keep the patient free of pain while the second is to fulfill the patient's emotional needs.

Pain relief at times can be difficult. As a physician, I had been taught to give the pain medication *after* the pain occurred for fear of giving the patient too much medication and causing an "addiction." This is the wrong approach with someone who has a terminal illness. Pain can be controlled by appropriate oral doses of narcotics given at regular intervals. The patient need not be confused by over-medication, and addiction in a terminal patient is the least of worries.

The loneliness of the last days, the fear of the unknown and the regret of goals not reached are problems that only family and friends can help resolve. Hospice Maui stands ready to help both the family and the patient during this difficult time.

Hospice Maui began its services in 1980 and has assisted hundreds of patients and families since that time. Presently, 45 patients are being aided with services of home visits by volunteers, with equipment loans to make home care easier, by visits of nurses specially trained in pain control, by assistance in coordinating community services, and by offering and giving help in any way that benefits the patient. Approximately 85% of Hospice Maui's patients are suffering from cancer. Another 10% have AIDS, while 5% have advanced cardiac (heart) or lung disease.

It is a credit to the community and to this wonderful organization that services so far have been provided free to the patient. This is possible because of wonderful volunteers and generous donations from the community. The first ten years of Hospice Maui's efforts have been outstanding, but the future is even more exciting. Their services will continue to expand along with Maui's growth, but the long term goal is building a Hospice facility which will have six to eight beds to care for patients who lack a family to help them. In their final days, Hospice Maui will become their family.

Bill, we will miss you. You showed the highest qualities of being a father, friend, community leader and attorney. We were all enriched by knowing you.

GENES AND THE FUTURE

Do you want to live a longer, healthier life? The answer is simple: "choose" your grandparents ver-r-ry carefully. If they lived to a "ripe old age" (whatever that means) and did not suffer from diabetes, cancer, rheumatoid arthritis, heart attacks or mental illnesses, then the chances are that you won't either. However, if you are like the rest of us, and have a family tree filled with these medical rotten apples, wouldn't you like to know that you are at risk so that you could do everything possible to avoid or minimize the potential illness? The cover story of the *U.S. News & World Report* (5-25-87) explains that in the future we may be able to do just that.

Our entire physical character, eye color, height, skin color, sex, etc..., and many of the illnesses which affect us through our lifetime, are determined by 23 pairs of chromosomes that we carry in each cell of our body. The chromosomes each contain thousands of "genes" which in turn are made up of complex molecules called DNA. Because of our grandparents' genes we are what we are, and we will pass these genes on to our children and grandchildren. Until recently, the chromosome puzzle was scientifically interesting, but not very practical, mostly because no one could break the code and discover what caused what. Today this view is changing rapidly.

Many Genetic Research Centers around the world have broken this DNA code, and the specific genes that cause many of our illnesses are being discovered weekly. By the year 2000 the "maps" of our chromosomes will have been printed, and it will be possible for an individual to obtain a genetic profile and "look into the future."

Geneticists at the University of Texas Health Science Center have discovered several mutant (not normal) genes which are involved in the premature onset of atherosclerosis (hardening of the arteries). These mutant genes cause heart attacks in people in their 30's. About one in 500 people have this "bad" gene. Another defective gene, discovered at Tufts University in Boston, may cause heart attacks after the age of 40. This gene interferes with the body's ability to produce HDL (high-density lipoprotein) that removes cholesterol from the bloodstream. Today there are about 12 genes known to play a part in the development of a heart attack. Because my mother, grandfather and uncle all died from heart attacks, I'm sure that I'm carrying around some of these genes. As a result I don't smoke, I avoid fatty foods and I exercise regularly. I hope that my efforts will prevent an early heart attack.

The study of cancer and genes is an exciting field and may someday lead to treatment or even prevention of this dreaded disease. So far, 36 human genes have been found to be involved with cancers. Ironically, these genes are also necessary for normal growth, so why do they go astray and cause a cancer in their host? At the University of Minnesota Medical School, researchers found that these oncogenes (cancer causing genes) were located near inherited weak points in the chromosomes. When the chromosome would break (because of x-rays, viruses or tobacco smoke) the rearrangement would expose the oncogene, and a cancer would start. The reason that some families do not have cancers is probably due to the fact that their chromosomes do not have "weak points." Thus, their oncogenes are never exposed, so a cancer never begins. Other families are not as fortunate, and many members may be afflicted with this disease. An exciting approach to cancer prevention will be finding drugs which will strengthen the "weak points" of our chromosomes and eliminate this danger.

The genetic study of mental illnesses has revealed many of them to be hereditary and offers the chance of early recognition. Huntington's disease (a severe progressive neurological illness) is always inherited and can now be recognized by a defective gene. The genes for dyslexia, Alzheimer's disease, manic depression and schizophrenia have been identified. There may even be a gene particular to alcoholics. Because some of these conditions are treatable, early recognition and medical help could minimize the condition.

The list of the ten genetic tests now available is impressive and includes the genes for adult polycystic kidney disease, sickle-cell anemia, cystic fibrosis, Huntington's disease and hemophilia. In the near future there will be genetic tests for dyslexia, arteriosclerosis, cancer, manic depression, schizophrenia, juvenile diabetes and multiple sclerosis. The only limit to the number of tests that can be developed may be the number of illnesses afflicting mankind.

So with all this information, what does the future hold? Was Aunt Tillie right when she said, "I told you not to marry Frank. All the members of his family that didn't die of cancer, went crazy." Will we try to "weed out" the bad apples? No, I believe that men and women will use their brains and build on this information. For example, gene-splicing is already being used with plants and animals. Genes are taken from one chromosome and placed into another to give the desired quality. I can envision "Gene-Banks" where healthy genes are available for replacement into defective chromosomes. If you had suffered from diabetes since childhood, wouldn't you like to protect your children and their children from the same fate?

Is this "playing God?" Perhaps, but we play God every time we get on an airplane and fly to Oahu or the Mainland. Some people insist that, "If God had meant us to fly he would have given us wings." Just as God gave us a brain to invent an airplane, He gave us a brain to discover how to decrease the pain and suffering of mankind. Let's use it.

SCARS

Have you had an operation and wondered why your scar was larger or smaller than your neighbor's, who had the same surgeon and procedure? Why are some scars so thin that they can hardly be seen while others are visible from across the room? There are several reasons. Hard as surgeons try, sometimes our beautiful incisions are rearranged by the body's methods of healing.

Collagen is the body's glue that bonds skin edges together. It is a protein that is secreted by fibroblast cells, special microscopic cells crucial in the healing of wounds. The more collagen secreted into an incision the thicker the scar. A perfect scar would have just the right amount of collagen to hold the skin together firmly, but not so much that a thickened scar forms. The body frequently continues producing collagen beyond the "glueing point" and it piles up into a thick, raised scar referred to by physicians as a "hypertrophic" scar.

There are several important rules surgeons have learned to reduce the number of hypertrophic or "thick" scars. If possible they try to make the incision in a skin crease. This is the reason that the incision for a thyroid operation is placed in one of the wrinkles running across the base of the neck. The incisions which leave the thinnest scars on the abdomen are those that are made from side to side. However, it is often necessary to make the incision "up and down" because more exposure is needed for the operation. In all cases,the success of an operation takes precedence over the appearance of the scar.

Other rules for reducing the incidence of hypertrophic scars include using fine sutures and avoiding infections. Even then, surgeons may be defeated.

The thickest, ugliest scars are called keloids. They may occur from only scratches and recur if they are excised. In the keloid the collagen is not only more abundant, but it also spreads beyond the boundaries of the incision. It is best to avoid elective or minor surgery on patients who form keloids.

The thick hypertrophic scars will slowly lose their redness and flatten out as the months pass by but will never become thinner.

The secret of a thin, almost invisible scar depends on the age of the patient. The older the patient, the more perfect the scar appears. This is because in later years there is less collagen deposited, and hence a thinner scar is formed. After putting the Medicare patients through the discomfort of major operations, it is comforting to know that they will have scars envied by their grandchildren.

SHOCK WAVES
FOR KIDNEY STONES

Star Wars in the body? The future is here! Lasers have been used for over ten years in eye surgery, and are now being used to blast through the blocked arteries of the legs and heart. But an exciting treatment, developed in the last few years, is using shock waves to destroy kidney stones.

Nine years ago, in Germany, "shock wave" therapy was used on the first kidney stone patient. The procedure is called extracorporeal (out of the body) shock wave lithotripsy (stone destruction), or ESWL for short. Shock waves are different from light waves or ultrasonic waves that have certain wavelengths with positive and negative deflections. A shock wave has a single positive pressure front that acts like a small hammer when it hits a stone. Fortunately, the shock wave passes through the skin, tissues and bone with little injury to these organs or little change in wave strength. If you were to take a piece of gravel from your driveway and hit it lightly with a hammer 1,000 to 2,000 times, the gravel would finally break down into little pieces of sand. This is what happens to the kidney stone during ESWL treatment.

The procedure is not painful, but the patient is first anesthetized because he must remain perfectly still for 30 to 45 minutes. Next, he is lowered into a stainless steel tub of warm water and positioned so that the stone, which is localized by x-ray, is at the point of maximum strength of the shock wave.

The shock waves are fired at about one second intervals, each one sounding much like a hammer hitting a nail. X-rays are taken of the kidney stone during the procedure until they show that the stone has been reduced to sand-like particles.

Frequently these particles will cause pain as they pass from the kidney to the bladder, and pain medications may be necessary during this period.

Often, the urologist will pass a tube from the bladder up to the kidney before the ESWL treatment. This tube assists in the passage of the sand, preventing the pain and possible obstruction of the ureter (the natural tube from the kidney to the bladder).

Has shock wave treatment been successful for kidney stones? Over 400,000 patients world-wide will answer "yes." The procedure is 99% successful for stones which are 3 cm. (1.2 inches) in size or smaller.

About 10% of patients will need a second procedure in order to clear the stone.

Hawaii has its own ESWL center in Honolulu. The Kidney Stone Center of the Pacific, although located at Queen's Hospital, is a joint venture of Queen's, Straub and Kuakini Hospitals. The cost of the treatment is about $6,000 to $7,000, about the same as for an operation. The advantages of ESWL treatment are several: avoiding an operation with its pain and possible complications, avoiding prolonged hospitalization, and returning to work and a normal life much sooner.

The FDA (Federal Drug Administration) has recently approved the investigation of ESWL treatment for gallstones in four research hospitals across the country. This certainly holds promise for the future, but gallstones are different from kidney stones. Frequently a patient with gallstones is critically ill from infection and needs immediate surgery. Moreover, not all gallstones respond to shock waves. Finally, the gallbladder will form the stones again if only the stones are removed. A patient can live a normal life without the gallbladder, which is not the case if his kidneys are removed.

Shock waves and lasers! What else will the medical care of the future hold for us? I can hardly wait!

EPIDERMAL CYSTS

Those unsightly cysts which people frequently get on their backs, faces or scalps—what are they? Are they dangerous? Can they turn into cancer?

A problem that I see almost daily in my office is a patient with an epidermal (skin) cyst. The cyst is lined with epidermis (that's how it got its name), which is actually the same covering as your outside skin. It occurs most commonly on the back, scalp, neck and face, although it can occur elsewhere on the body.

Other than being rather unattractive, a cyst is rarely dangerous; occasionally, however, it can become infected. This requires an incision and drainage of the pus that develops inside the cyst. The procedure is always done in the doctor's office and takes only a few minutes. Rarely do they become cancerous. In fact, I have not seen one change into a cancer in my 30 years of practice.

The most common problem is the unsightliness of the lump, and it is usually the nagging of the husband or wife that finally makes the spouse see the physician. The cyst can be removed as an office procedure, and the earlier one sees a physician the easier it is to remove. I believe the largest cyst that I have removed from the skin was 2 1/2 inches in diameter, which takes a longer time to remove and leaves a larger scar.

After the cyst is removed and cut open, the keratin material inside is cheese-like and very characteristic of the epidermal cyst.

Other lumps beneath the skin that can be confused with the epidermal cyst are lipomas (non-cancerous lumps of fat), neurofibromas (non-cancerous nerve tumors) and ganglions (cysts that arise from the joints, especially at the wrists.) Lumps and bumps beneath the skin are slightly disfiguring and rarely dangerous, but a visit to your physician will answer your questions and relieve your worries.

DOCTORS' NAMES

The medical profession has taken centuries to devise its vocabulary so that it will confuse patients who might be listening. We then hung titles on each other, depending upon one's specialty, so that a patient must now know Greek and Latin in order to understand exactly what the sign means on the doctor's door. Let me help you.

Your first lesson is in Greek. The suffix "logist" comes from the Greek word *logos*, meaning the study of a subject. So when we talk about gynecologists, urologists, pathologists or radiologists, we are talking about those doctors who have "studied" or specialized in particular fields of medicine. Now it becomes a little more complicated. Is a radiologist a doctor who studies radios? Or is a pathologist really a forest ranger who studies animal trails? What does a urologist study? Actually a general surgeon isn't a surgeon who operates only on generals, a plastic surgeon rarely uses plastic and a family practitioner is not really "practicing"—he knows what he is doing.

Here is a partial list of different specialties now available on Maui and the fields they encompass.

Although the term general surgery is used to include all fields of surgery, general surgeons spend most of their time caring for the problems of the abdomen, such as the stomach, gallbladder, hernias and intestine. They are also the first surgeons called for the treatment of an accident patient. They will then determine the need for other specialists such as orthopedic or neurosurgeons.

Obstetrics and gynecology (OB-GYN) includes the care of pregnant women, the delivery of children and the treatment of the many surgical and medical problems related to female organs.

Our friendly pediatricians, "baby doctors," are indispensable in the care of our youngsters, especially in critical diseases. They generally restrict their patients to those twelve or under in age.

An otorhinolaryngologist (how's that for a name?) is an ENT or ear, nose and throat specialist who takes care of all problems in these areas.

Ophthalmologists are eye specialists dealing not only in the refractions necessary for glasses, but also care for the serious medical and surgical problems of the eye.

Plastic surgeons try to improve on the work of God and do some beautiful work, but I have yet to meet one who can walk on water.

The urologist takes care of problems of the kidneys, urinary bladder and prostate gland.

Orthopedic surgeons (jokingly refered to as "bone pushers,") must "push" or rearrange the bones into their correct positions.

An internist is a physician who specializes in the care of patients with heart attacks, diabetes and other serious, non-surgical problems. Some internists will "sub-specialize" and limit their practice to gastroenterology (problems of the intestinal tract), oncology (the treatment of cancer patients requiring chemotherapy) or other fields.

The dermatologist is the one that patients seek out when they have skin rashes, itches, acne and unusual lumps and bumps of the skin.

Pathologists keep the rest of us on our toes by examining the tissues that we remove at surgery. They give us "the final diagnosis." They are also responsible for the modernization and updating of our laboratories which now can do hundreds of different tests on blood samples.

Radiologists, of course, do not repair radios. They "read" or interpret the x-rays and perform the numerous studies that are available and which have advanced medicine so greatly in the last 15 years.

The anesthesiologists have been nicknamed "gas passers" not because of their embarrassing habits, but because they frequently administer "gas" in order to put a patient to sleep for an operation.

Psychiatrists are referred to as "the shrinks," but the role they play in our modern society is vital in teaching us how to cope with our problems.

And last, but not least, is the backbone of good medical care, our family practitioner, who must understand and practice parts of all of the other specialties. He or she is the first line of medical care, the physician to whom the patient can turn for the initial examination.

Now that we all know "who's on first," I will ignore the humorous patient who asked, "Doctor, if you've been practicing for 25 years, when are you finally going to get it right?"

MEDICAL ORGANIZATIONS

MD, DO, FACS, FACP, FACOG.... What do all these initials mean after your doctor's name? How do these professional organizations help the physician or the patient?

MD is the abbreviation for the Latin words *Medicinae Doctor* and signifies that the individual is a doctor of "medicine" and has graduated from a medical school. DO means that the physician is a doctor of osteopathy, having graduated after four years at an osteopathic college. In addition to using the usual medical practices, he frequently uses manipulation in treating musculoskeletal problems.

When we talk of medical organizations, the "grand-daddy" of all is the American Medical Association, which is now 143 years old—or young—depending on your point of view. Since its founding in 1847, members have worked hard to follow its goal: "to promote the science and art of medicine and the betterment of public health." Over the years the AMA has had a long and impressive history of improving the health of our country. It established curriculum for medical schools and urged states to license only graduates of those schools as doctors (only 10% of doctors in 1847 were graduates). It helped states to register births, marriages and deaths. Nurse training programs, school hygiene, city water supply controls, milk quality standards, labeling of poisons, and the federal Food and Drug Administration are only a few of the hundreds of programs established by the AMA. Its 270,000 members (about 50% of the doctors in the country) are proud that their endeavors have given the American public the highest quality of medical care in the world!

As the doctors became more "specialized," they formed additional organizations to pursue their own interests in education and politics. There are now more than 200 organizations in this category. The American College of Surgeons is one of these.

In May of 1913, 500 prominent surgeons met in Washington, D.C. with the purpose of forming an association which would "benefit humanity by advancing the science of surgery." From this meeting has grown the American College of Surgeons which now has 50,000 members in the U.S. and Canada, and another 3,000 members from more than 100 other countries.

Through the years the ACS (American College of Surgeons) has established such programs as standards for hospitals, improving the training in surgical residency programs, establishing cancer and trauma programs in hospitals and a continuing education program to advance the surgical knowledge of its members.

It is not easy to become a fellow (member) of this association. Physicians must have completed an accepted surgical residency (four to six years of additional training after medical school) and have passed their specialty board examinations. Then after two years of practice in a community, they will be reviewed by the local chapter of the ACS as to their surgical skills and moral character before being recommended for membership. You can now appreciate why surgeons are so proud to have FACS (Fellow of the American College of Surgeons) after their MD.

In 1951, 11 obstetricians, realizing the need for improved OB care in the U.S., established the American College of Obstetricians and Gynecologists. Its membership has now grown to 26,000 members. Through their training programs and with increased technology and obstetrical care, the maternal mortality (mothers dying from child-birth) has decreased 91% and infant mortality (the infant dying at birth) has decreased 62% during the last 36 years. This is a record to be proud of.

The American Academy of Family Physicians has over 57,000 members and strives to "promote the science and art of medicine and surgery and the betterment of the public health and to preserve the patient's right to free choice of physician."

The American Academy of Orthopaedic Surgeons, the American Academy of Pediatrics, the American College of Emergency Physicians, the American College of Physicians (the organization for Internists), the American College of Radiologists and another hundred colleges, academies and associations have all been created for the specific purpose of educating their members. As a result, your doctors can keep abreast of the rapid changes in their fields of medicine and take better care of you and your loved ones. Moreover, America's high quality of medical care is due in large part to the vast amount of time and energies of these organizations in continuously educating their members.

MD, DO, FACS, FACP, FACOG, AMA...are now abbreviations that should carry some meaning for you.

Index

( )* Indicates articles in Two Aspirin – First Dose

128

ESWL   117
Eustachian tube   74
Fats
   monounsaturated   (17)*
   polyunsaturated   (17)*
   saturated   (17)*
Fever   47
Fiber   (72)*
Fiberscopes   (91-93)*
Fibroadenoma   88
Fish   (72)*
Fissure
   anal   (66)*
Fistula, anal   (66)*
Fitness   22
Fleming, Dr.   (7, 8)*
Florey, Dr.   (8)*
Fluoride   (60)*
Fox, Dr.   (12)*
Gallbladder   (65, 72-74)*
Ganglion   83, 119
Gas   63
Gastric bypass   (33)*
Gastritis   (6)*
Gastroscope   (69, 91)*
Genes   112
Goiter   84
Gout   65
Guaiac test   (37)*
Gynecologists   120
Gynecomastia   86
HDL   (16, 17, 22, 23)*
Head injury   (84)*
Heart attack   6, 48, 112, (6, 15, 22, 29, 64)*
Heart failure   (10)*
Hemorrhoids   (66)*
Hennekens, Dr. Charles   6
Hernia, inguinal   80, (74-76)*
Herpes
   simplex   (42)*
   zoster   (47)*
Hiatal hernia   (65)*
Hiccups   (62)*
High altitude illness   (60, 61)*

Hippocrates   47
HIV   (48)*
Hoarseness   53
Hodgkin's disease   (68)*
Hospice Maui   109
Hospice movement   109
Huntington's disease   113
Hypertension   92
Hyperthyroid   84
Hyperventilation   (63, 64)*
Hypocalcemia   (9)*
Hypothermia   102
Hypothyroid   84
Hypoxemia   67
Immune system   100
Inderal   56
Internist   121
Intestinal obstruction   78
ITP   100
Jellyfish   (31)*
Kennedy, President   (55)*
Kidney stones   117
Koop, Dr. C.E   (24, 52)*
Kowalski, Robert E.   (18, 20, 21, 23)*
Laryngitis   53
LDL   (16, 17, 22, 23)*
Lipomas   119
Lopid   (19)*
Lovastatin   (19)*
Lymph nodes   82, (67, 68)*
Lymphoma   (68)*
Mammograms   41
MASH   (86)*
Medical costs   (89, 90)*
Mesenteric adenitis   61
Metamucil   70
Mevacor   (19)*
Migraine headaches   55
Monosodium glutamate   55
Myocardial infarction   (64)*
Neck injuries   (31)*
Niacin   (22)*
Nicorettes   (27)*
Nicotine   16

( )* Indicates articles in Two Aspirin – First Dose

( )* Indicates articles in Two Aspirin – First Dose